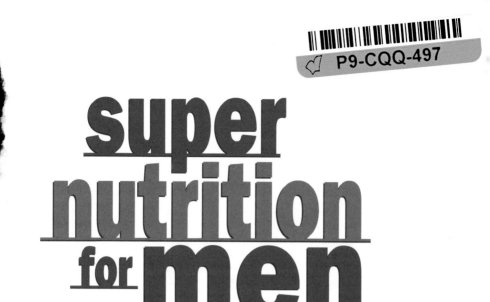

super
nutrition
for men

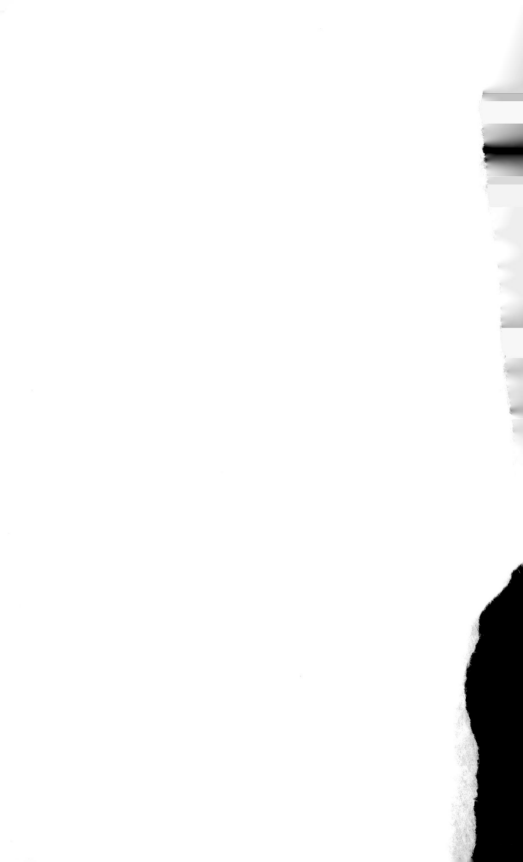

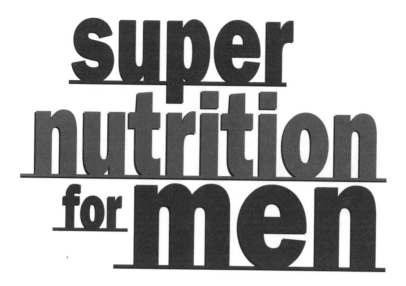

super nutrition for men

ann louise gittleman, MS, CNS

AVERY PUBLISHING GROUP

Garden City Park • New York

The nutritional, medical, and health information presented in this book is based on the training, personal experiences, and research of the author. It is intended for educational purposes, and is not meant to diagnose, prescribe, or replace medical care. Because each person and situation is unique, the author and publisher urge the reader to check with a qualified health professional before using any procedure where there is any question to appropriateness. The author and publisher are not responsible for any adverse effects or consequences from the use of the suggestions or procedures in this book.

The publisher does not advocate the use of any particular health care protocol, but believes the information presented in this book should be available to the public.

Cover Designer: Doug Brooks
In-House Editor: Peggy Hahn
Typesetter: Liz Johnson
Printer: Paragon Press, Honesdale, PA

Avery Publishing Group
120 Old Broadway
Garden City Park, NY 11040
1–800–548–5757
www.averypublishing.com

Cataloging-in-Publication Data

Gittleman, Ann Louise.
    Super nutrition for men / Ann Louise Gittleman.
  —1st ed.
    p. cm.
    Includes bibliographical references and index.
    ISBN: 0-89529-954-2

    1. Men—Nutrition. 2. Men—Health and hygiene.
  I. Title.

RA777.8.G58 1999   613.2'081
                                          QB199-739

Printed in the United States of America

10 9 8 7 6 5 4 3 2 1

Contents

This book is lovingly dedicated to my father,
Arthur Gittleman — the first man in my life.

Acknowledgments

First and foremost my greatest thanks to Susan Stockton, my right hand, and to Carol Faye Templeton, my brilliant little computer whiz.

I also owe a lot to the men in my life.

There have been many male role models whom I have learned from since I was a little girl, including my father and my brother, Stuart. So what better way to recognize them than in a book dedicated to the good health and longevity of men?

To Aaron Kriwitsky—my grandfather—a religious scholar who taught me the holiness of the written and spoken word.

To Rabbi Haskel Lindenthal—my religious school mentor—who cultivated in me the value of learning and study.

To Emerich Ohlbaum—one of my Dad's closest friends—whose amazing work ethic and lively personality never ceased to amaze me.

To John Harris—my high school English teacher—whose voice I still hear in my head as I compose my manuscripts.

To Edward Aldworth—a truly elegant gentleman who is both kind and shrewd.

To Chuck Kambourian—the most talented and devoted family man I know.

To Don Meredith—a living legend who is as charming in real life as he was on Monday night football.

To Chuck Diker—a great business leader and humanitarian.

To Jeff Howard—a man whose integrity and forward thinking I greatly admire.

To John Desgrey—a man who taught me how to visualize and make dreams come true.

And to all the other great guys who have contributed to my life in their own way. Here's to Josh Rubenstein, my dear childhood friend who went on to become a writer and spokesperson for the political prisoners of the world; to Paul Kimatian, a talented producer who taught me "how to do lunch" and guided me during my years in California; and to James William Templeton who has made my life complete.

1.

Putting the Power of Nutrition to Work for You

L ike winning the lottery, this book will change your life. If you're tired of diet and exercise programs that just don't work, and you can use some practical advice on staying fit, enhancing your sex life, overcoming an addiction, or protecting your heart and prostate naturally, then this book is for you. *Super Nutrition for Men,* based on cutting-edge research and my own clinical experience over twenty years, is for men from eighteen to eighty.

Within these first few chapters, you'll discover how cutting down on carbohydrates and increasing your intake of the right fats will turn your body into a fat-burning machine. You'll learn about the latest wave in getting fit fast—the 40/30/30 plan—used by world-class athletes to significantly improve athletic performance and recovery from exercise. The good news about the 40/30/30 plan is that it allows even the couch potato to use stored body fat for fuel. This plan helps boost energy, improve concentration and attention span, increase lean muscle mass, and curb food cravings.

In reading this book, you'll begin to look at food from a whole new perspective—as fuel for both the body and the mind. You will learn how food affects hormone levels, and how the right foods can positively impact peak performance, mood, and overall health.

Outlined in these pages are many innovative programs for protecting your prostate, healing your heart, super-charging sex, reducing hair loss, overcoming addictions, and eating right—at home and on the go. All of these programs can fit into busy schedules. Most of them require minor adjustments in the way you live. Some may not be quite as simple, but the rewards will be worth the effort!

Super Nutrition for Men is a no-nonsense handbook that contains answers to the questions most frequently asked by my male clients, such as:

- Is it really possible to avoid prostate problems?

- Can I still eat healthy if I'm a meat and potatoes man?

- If heart disease runs in the family, are there natural therapies I can use to prevent it?

- Is there anything I can do about my thinning hair?

- Are there any secrets I should know that can help me improve my sex life?

- What's the latest on drugless treatments to get off caffeine and nicotine? How about marijuana and cocaine?

This book is unique, different than anything you've ever read before on men's health. *Super Nutrition for Men* gives you up-to-the-minute health and nutrition strategies. You will learn all the formulas for staying on top—formulas that you haven't read about in any other books or magazine articles, or seen on TV. And the programs I suggest are derived from the research of some of the most respected authorities around the world.

And, by the way, this book is not just for men. It's for the women who love them. So, don't be afraid to have your wife, girlfriend, or significant other peruse these pages with you. Better still, buy her a copy.

WHERE MEN STAND

Here are the real life, hard-core statistics and data that compelled me to write *Super Nutrition for Men.* Men lead in eight of the ten top causes of death in the United States. They are generally reluctant to seek medical care, and when they finally do decide to see a physician, their illnesses have often progressed to a more critical state.

Although heart disease remains the number one killer among men, only one-third of those in the forty-five to sixty-four age group have ever had their cholesterol levels checked. Among men over fifty, only one out of two knows the warning signs of prostate or colorectal cancer, and one out of five reports being too embarrassed to discuss the matter with his doctor. A mere 22 percent of men over forty report having had a digital rectal exam (DRE) to check for prostate problems in the previous year, despite the fact that annual DRE exams are recommended by authorities for all middle-aged men.

Men are equally reluctant to seek counseling and emotional support, and they constitute only 30 percent of the patients who consult psychologists and psychiatrists. This is despite the fact that men commit over 90 percent of violent crime, abuse alcohol and drugs three times as much as women do, and commit suicide three times as often.

Obesity

While men are far less likely to go on diets or join weight-loss programs, they're no less likely to be overweight. In fact, statistics reveal that more American men are obese than are American women—26.1 percent compared with 25.1 percent. Maybe this has something to do with the fact that only 47 percent of men pay attention to food's nutritional content.

Male pattern obesity, in which weight is concentrated in the middle of the body, is more dangerous than female pattern obesity because it increases the risk of developing cardiovascular disease. Obesity is also a risk factor for diabetes and is linked to the development of certain forms of cancer, gall bladder disease, hypertension, musculoskeletal problems, sleep apnea, and stroke. According to Dr. Morton Shaevitz, Director of Eating Disorders Programs at Scripps Clinic and Research Foundation, the bottom line is that "fat men die young."

And yet, men lose weight more easily than women for reasons that are largely physiological. While men are less likely to take overt steps to control their weight, there's strong evidence that they do care about their appearance, and a growing number are choosing to have aesthetic, or plastic, surgery. Over the past twenty-five years, 30 percent of such surgeries have been performed on men. Procedures commonly sought by men include liposuction, eyelid surgery, rhinoplasty (nose job), and face lift.

The good news is that losing weight and keeping it off will increase longevity. In fact, losing only 10 percent or less of body weight can increase life span, and substantially improve hypertension, adult onset diabetes, and cardiovascular disease. And, although men may dislike the idea of dieting, they're good at losing weight when they resolve to do so.

Stress

One of the biggest problems with the Standard American Diet (SAD) is that it stresses the body. It acts as a stressor because it depletes nutrient reserves, which in turn decreases the body's ability to handle stress. Stress contributes to increased rates of fatigue, heart attacks, and hypertension among males. This is a special problem for men, who are more susceptible to stress-related disorders, due to their tendency to hold feelings in and deny problems, and their reluctance to admit setbacks.

Poor diet, eating on-the-go, overwork, lack of exercise, and family responsibilities are just a few of the stressors present in the life of today's man. Others include use of tobacco, alcohol, steroids, antibiotics, and other chemical substances. These elements contribute to nutrient depletion, putting more stress upon the body and decreasing the body's coping ability. Fortunately, this vicious cycle can be broken with good nutrition.

THE DIFFERENCE MARRIAGE MAKES

Odds are six to one that a husband will die before his wife, though married men will likely fare better than single men. In fact, single men and widowers suffer more heart attacks and, overall, their life spans are shorter. Plus, their suicide rate is triple that of married men.

Perhaps the primary health benefit that men reap from marriage has to do with the nurturing they receive. The female customarily assumes a nurturing role, which literally involves providing nourishment for her family. It has traditionally been held that it's a woman's job to know about food and its selection and preparation. And, of course, in the 1990s the link between diet and health is well established.

Women also provide necessary emotional nurturing. They tend to worry about their husbands. While a single man may ignore a health problem and put off medical consultation, a married man will likely seek medical advice sooner with some prompting from his spouse.

INTERPRETING MISGUIDED NUTRITIONAL MESSAGES

In April of 1992, the United States Department of Agriculture (USDA) adopted the Food Guide Pyramid as a replacement for the traditional four food groups that we all learned about in elementary school. The new guide recommends that carbohydrates—particularly bread, cereal, rice, and pasta—become the main focus of meals. Proteins like meat, fish, beans, and eggs are more of an accompaniment, not the main foundation. Fats, oils, and sweets are on the top of the pyramid, indicating that we need to cut way back on these foods. *Super Nutrition for Men* will show you how this kind of misguided information can exact a heavy toll, because certain kinds of fats are absolutely essential for prostate and heart health, and—believe it or not—for weight control, as well. Unfortunately, this lopsided view of healthy eating presented by the Food Guide Pyramid has perpetuated the high-carbohydrate craze that is directly related to America's growing pot belly.

GET READY TO TAKE UP THE CHALLENGE

These days, more men are actively seeking to improve their health with proper nutrition. Not only is nutrition a potent weapon for preventing disease and extending life span, it's also an excellent tool for achieving overall wellness. But the real challenge in our "Information Age" is one of wading through tons of nutrition books with diametrically opposed philosophies on how to achieve good nutrition, sorting it all out, and then finding a simple way to make practical use of the newly found information. Needless to say, this can be difficult, time-consuming, and confusing.

Applying the no-hassle health and nutrition guidelines in this book may take away the confusion, but will require motivation and commitment. I remember reading the words of a physician, writing about men's health issues, who stated that he is typically harder on men than on women. His approach works, he says, because approached honestly, men will take up a challenge. Consider *Super Nutrition for Men* as an open invitation to take up the challenge and take charge of the lifestyle modifications that will change and maybe even save your life.

2.

Lean and Mean: Cut the Carbs, Add the Fat

O ver the last decade, expert advice has directed us to boost our intake of carbohydrates and dramatically decrease our consumption of fats. During that time, the average weight of Americans has increased by ten pounds. Nonetheless, the "eat more/weigh less" mantra continues to echo through our homes, offices, and gyms. It has led to excessively high-carbohydrate diets, with sometimes as much as 70 percent of calories coming from carbohydrates. While this type of diet may work for some men, it will more than likely lead the majority not only into a condition of overweight, but also one of blood sugar instability that can sap vital energy and dull the mind. No one diet will work for all men all of the time simply because everyone is biochemically unique. That uniqueness is shaped by ancestry, genetic heritage, and metabolic rate, all of which must be taken into consideration in personalizing a diet plan.

Every man wants to be strong and solid, and most believe that the best way to achieve an ideal body is through exercise. Although exercise has numerous benefits and is indeed an essential tool in body shaping, you may be surprised to learn that diet is equally important for two reasons. First, food consumption triggers the release of hormones that determine whether we will store excess body fat or burn it. Second, due to their hormonal effect, food choices can reduce or enhance the benefits of exercise.

This chapter will introduce you to a diet plan that works for most men most of the time and can be modified to meet individual needs. The formula is a special balance of fats, carbohydrates, and protein designed to switch the body into a fat-burning mode. It calls for 40 percent of total calories to be derived from carbohydrates (like bread, pasta, and potatoes), 30 percent from natural and unprocessed fats (such as butter and olive oil), and 30 percent from protein (including low-fat cottage cheese, turkey, water-packed tuna, eggs, fish, chicken, and lean beef). Many men can expect to increase lean muscle mass on this program in as little as thirty days, while trimming body fat to the ideal range of 14 to 18 percent.

The 40/30/30 diet plan was pioneered by Barry Sears, Ph.D., formerly of the Boston School of Medicine and Massachusetts Institute of Technology. Independent studies from Pepperdine University and Sansum Medical Research Foundation in Santa Barbara, California have demonstrated that the 40/30/30 formula not only improves athletic performance significantly, but raises the level of the "good" HDL cholesterol and aids in weight loss. This program is also safe and effective for people with diabetes.

Research conducted over the last thirty years has shown that the proportions of the basic nutrients—carbohydrate, fat, and protein—determines whether we store fat or burn it. With the right mix of these nutrients, your body can become a fat-burning machine.

THE ROLE OF CARBOHYDRATES

The primary role of carbohydrates is to supply the energy that your body needs to function each day. Carbohydrates are abundant in plant foods, such as fruits, vegetables, peas, and beans. In general, foods derived from animals are not known to be rich in carbohydrates, although milk and milk products do contain significant amounts.

Carbohydrates are divided into two groups—simple carbohydrates and complex carbohydrates. *Simple carbohydrates,* including glucose and fructose, are found in sugar and fruits, and are readily digested. *Complex carbohydrates* are found in vegetables, as well as whole grains, beans, and legumes. These carbohydrates are called starches, and are also made up of sugars, but the sugar molecules are strung together to make up long, complex chains. Therefore, starch provides the body with a slow, steady supply of glucose because it must first be broken down during digestion.

Through digestion and metabolism, carbohydrates are converted into glucose, or blood sugar, to be used for fuel. The glucose is either used directly to provide energy for the body, or stored in the liver for future use.

Carbohydrate Overloading

While carbohydrate consumption may have the *immediate* effect of increasing energy by raising blood sugar, the long-term result of overconsumption will be the lowering of sugar levels. Carbohydrate overload most often takes the form of excessive consumption of grains, especially wheat. In the short-term, overload results in fatigue that is characteristic of low blood sugar, or *hypoglycemia.* The ultimate consequence, however, may be the development of a more severe blood-sugar disorder such as diabetes. In fact, the incidence of type II adult onset diabetes has increased alarmingly in recent years, especially among black and Hispanic people. Over 6 million American men now suffer from diabetes, while an estimated 3 million have early signs of the disease. Clearly, America has been growing sick and tired—and fat—as a result of the low-fat, high-carbohydrate craze.

Evidence suggests that prior to the agricultural revolution, some ten thousand years ago, our ancestors subsisted on a diet approximating the macronutrient ratio of the 40/30/30 plan. They did not eat grains or dairy products. But changes in our diet have outpaced genetic adaptations. Our digestive systems have not evolved sufficiently to accommodate the incorporation of large amounts of grain. Wheat represents over 80 percent of our total grain consumption. Gluten, a plant protein found in wheat, rye, oats, and barley is not handled well by an increasing number of individuals. Though heredity plays a role in "gluten intolerance" (also known as sprue or celiac disease), diet is the initiating factor.

In gluten-sensitive individuals, the plant protein damages the lining of the intestines, causing malabsorption. The body's inability to fully utilize vitamins and minerals leads to the development of any of the following symptoms: anemia, bloating, bone or joint pain, diarrhea, headache, intestinal pain, and muscle spasms and cramps. Gluten-intolerant men can substitute grains such as rice, millet, and buckwheat.

Another problem with grains—especially wheat, rye, and oats—is their high phytic-acid content. Phytic acid, a phosphorus-like compound, interferes with calcium absorption and limits absorption of other essential minerals, including iron, magnesium, and zinc. It's concentrated in grain husks, so even healthy whole grains can provide high levels of phytic acid due to their bran content. Commercial breads also contain this compound in their yeast.

Overconsumption of carbohydrates, paired with underconsumption of essential fats, contributes to the proliferation of the yeast germ *Candida albicans,* and to the development of hypothyroidism and adrenal insufficiency. These are all common conditions today that can lead to food allergies and sugar cravings. These conditions, in turn, aggravate the problem by depressing the body's ability to metabolize carbohydrates.

The Insulin Response

Hormonal balance is a key to health maintenance and/or restoration. Since food elicits hormonal responses that can be beneficial or detrimental, it's a good idea to cultivate the habit of conscious eating. We need to be aware of the effect our food choices will have—not only on our health, but on our appearance and mental state as well.

Losing weight on the high-carbohydrate diet can be difficult for some men, and keeping it off may be even harder. The unsuspected key to successful fat-burning is the hormone insulin. And insulin levels are controlled by the amount of carbohydrate in the diet. When we consume carbohydrates, the pancreas secretes insulin, which makes it possible for glucose, or blood sugar, to enter the cells and be converted into energy. Insulin prevents blood sugar from rising too high after a meal. It is a storage hormone that's responsible for storing excess blood sugar as glycogen in the liver and muscle tissues. Glycogen storage capacity is limited. Once it's exhausted, the body will convert excess carbohydrate to fat and store it under the direction of insulin.

Insulin is one of two hormones that is critically important to blood sugar control. The other, called *glucagon*, is released in response to protein consumption. Glucagon's action is the opposite to that of insulin. They are inversely paired hormones—when one is high, the other is low. Glucagon is a mobilization hormone. When blood-sugar level drops—and with it, energy level—glucagon is secreted by the pancreas, causing stored sugar (glycogen) to be released as glucose from the liver to replenish the sugar supply in the blood. Glucagon release also raises energy levels by increasing the release of fatty acids from fat cells. So, while insulin lowers blood sugar and stores fat, glucagon raises blood sugar and mobilizes fat from storage. Obviously, too much insulin will sap energy and increase body fat.

Carbohydrate overloading tends to displace proteins needed by the body for immunity, stable blood-sugar levels, hormones, and tissue repair. Additionally, carbohydrates such as bread, pasta, and potatoes are deficient in essential fats needed for the production of fat-burning hormones known as eicosanoids. The overconsumption of carbohydrates, with its subsequent stimulation of the insulin response, can lead to such effects as bloating, cardiovascular disease, fatigue, food cravings, and weight gain.

Many people consume complex carbohydrates in hopes of stabilizing blood sugar. What they are not aware of, however, is that some complex carbohydrates have a very high *glycemic index*, which means that they convert quickly to blood sugar and therefore raise insulin levels rapidly. The glycemic index is a measure of the effect of carbohydrate on blood glucose levels. It compares how rapidly carbohydrates are converted to blood sugar compared with glucose, which is given an index of 100. (See Chapter 12 for more detailed information about the glycemic index.)

FAT PHOBIA

Fat phobia gave birth to the carbohydrate craze that has by no means been limited to athletes. Fat-phobic individuals are everywhere. They're often motivated by a desire to lose weight and decrease the risk of developing the number-one killer in this country, heart disease. Many of these individuals avoid such basic nutritional staples as meat, eggs, and butter due to erroneous information they've received about cholesterol and fat. Instead, they fill up on sugar, which, ironically, will cause them to gain added pounds and increase their risk of developing cardiovascular disease.

The truth is that some amount of dietary fat is essential for good health. Besides providing insulation, which helps to maintain body temperature, fat acts as protective padding for your bones and internal organs. Fats facilitate oxygen transport, and are required for hormone production. They also aid in the absorption of the fat-soluble vitamins A, D, E, and K, and nourish the skin, mucous membranes, and nerves. And fats known as *phospholipids* are components of all cell membranes and other cellular structures. Without fat in your body, your cell membranes and nervous system would collapse. You would not be able to survive.

Of course, it's possible to overdo fat consumption, and many Americans do. As nutritionist Robert Crayhon, puts it: "Too much fat is a problem, but so is too much brown rice, exercise, or water. Anything in excess is unhealthy."[1] And regardless of the quantity of fat consumed, if the quality is poor, health problems will develop. Poor quality fat includes fats and oils that have had the "good" fat refined right out of them.

The typical American diet includes too much total fat, too much of the wrong kinds of fats, and too little of the right kinds. But the opposite extreme, a diet very low in fat, can cause problems, too. Let's take a look at some of the different types of fats, and how they affect the body.

Classification of Fats

Fats are composed of building blocks called *fatty acids.* There are three major types of fatty acids found in the diet and in the body: saturated, polyunsaturated, and monounsaturated. These chemical terms relate to the type and number of hydrogen bonds in the chemical structure of the fatty acid. The three different types of fatty acids have distinct characteristics and are predominant in different foods.

Saturated fatty acids (SFAs) have straight molecules, and they tend to be solid at room temperature. SFAs are found mainly in animal products, including meat fats, dairy products, coconut oil, cocoa butter, palm oil, and palm-kernel oil. Saturated fats have gotten the reputation of being "bad" fats because of their connection with high cholesterol and hardening of the arteries, but they are not bad in and of themselves. Moderate amounts of saturated fats, when consumed in balance with the essential fatty acids and a full spectrum of other nutrients, are not problematic in a healthy body. Too much saturated fat in the bloodstream, however, can prevent the blood from supplying sufficient amounts of the healthy essential fatty acids to the organs that need them.

Monounsaturated fatty acids (kernel) have one kink or bend in their molecules. They are liquid at room temperature, but solid when refrigerated. Oils such as olive, almond, apricot, kernel, peanut, canola (rapeseed), high-oleic safflower, and high-oleic sunflower oils are all monounsaturated fatty acids.

Polyunsaturated fatty acids (PUFAs) have two or more kinks in their molecules. These fats remain liquid even when refrigerated, and can be found in corn, soybean, safflower, and sunflower oils. The omega-3 and omega-6 essential fatty acids, which we will discuss next, are polyunsaturated fatty acids.

Essential Fatty Acids

Essential fatty acids (EFAs) are necessary for life and health. These fatty acids cannot be made by the body, so they must be supplied by the diet. Omega-3 and omega-6 fats are the two EFAs that we require for good health, and omitting them from the diet can result in serious health problems.

Your body uses essential fatty acids to rebuild and produce new cells, and to maintain proper brain and nervous-system function. EFAs also help transport "bad" fats out of the body by emulsifying and moving saturated fats and cholesterol through the bloodstream and out of artery and tissue deposits. In addition, these fats control the cardiovascular and reproductive systems, and are crucial to the functioning of the immune system. Without EFAs, cell membranes weaken, making the body vulnerable to infection. Finally, essential fatty acids are also believed to have enzymelike functions or to be cofactors in enzymes.

Animal studies have shown that deficiencies in essential fatty acids can result in eczema and sterility. A deficiency of these essential fats can also cause acne; arthritis; dry, flaky skin; and inflammation. Overweight is linked with EFA deficiency as well, since, in the absence of essential fatty acids, the body converts sugar to fat much more rapidly. This causes blood sugar to drop and appetite to increase, giving rise to overeating.

Recent research has found that over 20 percent of adults, as well as many children and infants, have abnormally low levels of omega-3 fatty acids. Studies have shown that people on extreme fat-restricted diets can show very low levels of omega-3s—less than 5 percent of normal in some cases. Worse still, illness creates a dramatically increased need for these EFAs. The following is a list of conditions known to correlate with omega-3 deficiencies. It was compiled by Dr. Bruce West and appeared in the March 1995 edition of his *Health Alert* newsletter:

- AIDS
- Alcoholism
- B-vitamin deficiencies
- Cirrhosis
- Coronary artery disease

- Coronary occlusion
- Crohn's disease
- Kidney disease
- Lupus
- Multiple sclerosis

- Obesity
- Sepsis (infection)
- Retinitis pigmentosa
- Sjogren-Larsen syndrome
- Reye's syndrome
- Skin disease
- Rheumatoid arthritis
- Vitamin-E deficiency
- Scleroderma
- Wiscott-Aldrich syndrome

Flaxseed oil is the best vegetable source of the omega-3s. Its consumption helps to oxygenate the body. It can be used liberally in salad dressings and/or substituted for butter over vegetables and grains. However, it cannot be used for cooking, as it is very heat sensitive. Canola oil, a monounsaturated oil, is another good vegetable source of omega-3 fatty acids. It was developed in Canada from the rapeseed plant. Canola oil has a mild taste and may be used on salads, for baking, and for low-heat recipes. Other sources of omega-3 linolenic acid include cold-water fish—salmon, mackerel, sardines, tuna, herring, and anchovies—wild game, flax oil, walnuts, pumpkin seeds, chia seeds, soybeans, wheat sprouts, fresh sea vegetables, and leafy greens. Omega-6 linoleic acid can be found in vegetable oils, legumes, all nuts and seeds, most grains, organ meats, lean meats, leafy greens, borage, evening primrose oil, and gooseberry and black currant oils.

While no one knows the exact amount of omega-3 and omega-6 fats needed for optimal health, researchers are warning us to be careful to maintain a good balance of these EFAs. A healthy ratio is said to be no more than three times more omega-6 than omega-3 fatty acids. High levels of omega-6 fatty acids, out of balance with the omega-3s, can promote health problems. For example, consuming too many omega-6 fats in relationship to omega-3s over a period of time will increase the risk of developing inflammatory and degenerative disorders like arthritis, urinary tract disorders, coronary artery disease, lupus, or multiple sclerosis. We can correct this imbalance by adding more omega-3s from the food sources listed above. However, we must be careful not to overcorrect the initial problem, because an overabundance of omega-3s can cause excessive bleeding, whereas omega-3 deficiency can lead to excessive clotting and artery obstruction. The higher the ratio of omega-3 to omega-6 fatty acids, the less likely that a clot will obstruct the artery.

Replacing saturated fat with essential fats will lead to a healthier, leaner body. EFAs are burned up in the body faster than other dietary fats and their presence is vital in the diet to achieve weight loss. One omega-6 EFA in particular, gamma-linolenic acid (GLA), activates the fat-burning process.

> *Jeff, a forty-two-year-old overweight male who believed he was doing everything right could not lose a pound. He had read "Beyond Pritikin" and called my office to inquire whether he, a male could go on the same program as his wife. She was following a lower carbohydrate diet and adding GLA in the form of evening primrose oil to her regimen. She not only lost her desired seven pounds, but also several inches around her waist. I encouraged Jeff to follow a similar program and get on the GLA pronto. Three weeks later Jeff wired a dozen roses to the office with a note: "Thanks—One rose for every pound lost."*

Omega-3s actually lower triglycerides and the level of "bad" LDL cholesterol in the body. Adults need a total intake of two to five tablespoons of EFA-rich oil daily. Most of this amount can be obtained from food—whole foods, not refined ones. Generally, I recommend supplemental amounts of EFAs—one tablespoon of flaxseed oil per day for the omega-3 it provides, and one tablespoon of unrefined safflower oil or four capsules of GLA from evening primrose oil as a source of omega-6 EFAs.

Fat-Burning Friends

While carbohydrate consumption raises insulin levels and lowers glucagon, protein consumption does the opposite—it raises glucagon and lowers insulin. This is where the need for macronutrient balance comes into play. Fats enter the picture in that they affect the production of a little known group of hormones called *eicosanoids*. Though their importance has been recognized only recently, eicosanoids are the oldest known hormones and, like glucagon, they are fat-burning friends when the right kind are released. They are said to act only upon the cell that produces them or upon an adjacent cell and are known to exist for only a few seconds.

Therefore, unlike the many other hormones, eicosanoids cannot be measured. They are a part of natural body chemicals with such exotic names as leukotrienes, thromboxanes, and prostaglandins. These substances regulate every cell in the body and are essential to every life form on the planet. Eicosanoids are made from linoleic acid, one of the EFAs. It is not just EFA intake however, but everything else that is eaten as well, that will determine the amounts and ratios of the different kinds of eicosanoids generated from the linoleic acid. Simply stated, there are "good" series-1 and "bad" series-2 eicosanoids. The functions of these hormones are summarized in Table 2.1 on page 18.

Good eicosanoids regulate the cardiovascular system and control the mobilization of stored body fat. The balance of macronutrients in the diet will determine the ratio of good-to-bad eicosanoids. An excess of series-2 eicosanoids can lead to:

- Allergies
- Asthma
- Atherosclerosis
- Autoimmune diseases
- Cancer
- Connective tissue disease
- Fluid retention
- Heart attack
- High blood pressure
- Infections
- Pulmonary embolism
- Stroke
- Thrombophlebitis

In fact, every known symptom and disease process requires an excess of series-2 eicosanoids.[2] The most important dietary factor in determining a favorable eicosanoid balance is protein-to-carbohydrate ratio. Overproduction of series-2 eicosanoids results from excessive carbohydrate intake and inadequate intake of dietary protein. According to research, the ideal ratios are reflected in the

Table 2.1. The Opposing Functions of Eicosanoids

"Good" Series-1 Eicosanoids	"Bad" Series-2 Eicosanoids
Dilate blood vessels	Constrict blood vessels
Anti-clotting	Clot forming
Bronchial dilatation	Bronchial constriction
Control cell proliferation	Increase cell proliferation
Strengthen immunity	Weaken immunity
Anti-inflammatory	Pro-inflammatory
Reduce cholesterol synthesis	Increase cholesterol synthesis
Decrease pain	Increase pain

40/30/30 formula. A significant alteration of these percentages at any meal can throw off hormonal balance. And, if carbohydrate levels are too high, body fat will be stored and blood sugar lowered.

Jay Robb, a California-based fitness consultant and author of *The Fat Burning Diet* (Loving Health Publications, 1994), knows first-hand about the problems associated with a low-fat, high-carbohydrate diet and the advantages gained from cutting carbohydrates and adding fat. Robb spent sixteen years searching for the perfect diet to control his hypoglycemia. Through trial and error, he hit upon a diet plan that not only controls blood sugar, but also assists in fat-burning. He now advocates a diet that is low in natural carbohydrates and contains adequate protein and healthy fat. According to Robb: "The body is designed to use carbohydrates as fuel only temporarily. When we return to natural fat burning—which is what you're doing before you have that cereal and fruit for breakfast—all insulin is controlled."[3]

Also in the eicosanoid category are hormones called *prostaglandins*. These are involved in such vital processes as blood clotting, hormone production, inflammation, pain perception, and smooth muscle contraction. As members of the eicosanoid family, there are "good" and "bad" prostaglandins. The balance of omega-6 to omega-3 oils is critical to proper prostaglandin metabolism.

Unfortunately, this balance is upset in the Standard American Diet (SAD), which is composed largely of processed foods from which omega-3s have been removed to retard spoilage. Our diets also tend to be deficient in EPA, an omega-3 fatty acid found in cold-water fish, wild game, and flaxseed and canola oils. Deficiency of this fatty acid is also intensified by consumption of hydrogenated fats that produce the bad prostaglandins. (Hydrogenation will be discussed in greater detail in Chapter 3.)

40/30/30 BALANCE FOR ATHLETIC PERFORMANCE

With today's emphasis on carbohydrate loading for athletes, a typical diet often consists of 70-percent carbohydrate, 15-percent protein, and 15-percent fat. This kind of fuel mix elevates insulin levels, encouraging hypoglycemia with an accompanying lack of concentration. Fat is stored and any of the health problems associated with unfavorable eicosanoid production can develop. Such effects obviously impair athletic performance and provide the biochemical scenario for the marathon runner who hits the wall or the tennis player who loses his focus after a few hours.

The more desirable 40/30/30 balance of macronutrients allows the body to access its primary source of muscle energy, fatty acids, which are stored in adipose tissue (body fat). On a high-carbohydrate diet, this stored fat is not easily accessed, and the muscles instead use carbohydrates, an inferior fuel, as a source of energy. According to Dr. Philip Maffetone, applied kinesiologist and trainer/coach for professional athletes, fat provides over twice the energy of carbohydrates—nine calories per gram, as opposed to four calories per gram in carbohydrates. Dr. Maffetone believes that athletes are missing the boat with their high-carbohydrate intake: "The average U.S. athlete has a career span of four and a half years. . . . This is what happens when you rely on your sugar reserves, not fat reserves."[4]

When Maffetone first began working with Mark Allen, the Iron Man Champion was running a 7-minute mile. Eleven years later he was doing 5:10-minute miles and doing them at a lower heart rate. During this period of time, the athlete actually became physiologically "younger," according to Maffetone. Allen credits these re-markable results to the way he trains and the 40/30/30 eating plan.

The higher proportion of energy obtained from fat with the 40/30/30 balance of macronutrients results in the conservation of muscle glycogen that keeps blood-sugar levels elevated, im-proving the athlete's concentration, focus, and endurance. The 40/30/30 diet can also help to:

- Decrease hunger
- Enhance cardiovascular endurance
- Improve memory and mental alertness

- Increase fat burning
- Increase lean body mass
- Reduce fatigue

Many of the beneficial effects are attributed to the release of growth hormone from the pituitary gland that is stimulated by good (series-1) eicosanoids. Growth hormone builds and repairs muscle tissue.

Since the benefits of the 40/30/30 approach to macronutrient balance were initially determined through studies with athletes, the area of sports nutrition has been the first to make practical applica-tion of the principles. The Balance Bar Company has sponsored studies showing the efficacy of this approach to eating and they have developed a tasty nutrition bar appropriately named Balance.* Formulated according to the 40/30/30 ratio of macronutrients, it is a definite contrast to most sports and energy bars that usually con-tain 75- to 90-percent carbohydrates. Balance bars can be used as a meal replacement, though they should not substitute for more than one meal a day. They also provide good appetite control—three to five hours for most people—and only 180 calories.

ACHIEVING BALANCE

By now it should be clear that conditions of imbalance on both the chemical and energetic levels create fatigue, weight problems, and disease. Achieving hormonal balance by eating properly allows us

---

* The Balance nutrition bar is available through The Balance Bar Company (1–800–678–4246).

to regain health and achieve our genetic weight. The 40/30/30 eating plan is designed to re-establish this balance and it will no doubt work wonders for many people—perhaps even the majority of those who try the plan. Let us bear in mind, however, that studies demonstrating its efficacy were primarily conducted with athletes, so we may not be able to generalize the results to the general public. In truth, I believe that there really is no one diet that is best for all people.

While I've been pretty hard on the low-fat, high-carbohydrate diet as a panacea for every man, I must admit that it may be therapeutic for some, at least in the short run. However, I do believe that for others, the net results will be counterproductive for the reasons outlined in the previous pages. Just as a diet too heavy on carbohydrates can be deleterious to the health, so can one too high in proteins or too high in fats. Balance is the key. However, what puts one man in balance might throw another off because of biochemical individuality.

The Pritikin diet, which is very high in complex carbohydrates and low in fat and protein, has had its success stories. So has the Atkins diet, which is very low in complex carbohydrates, but high in protein. These radically different diets both have had beneficial results—but not with the same people. So what are the factors that determine the type of diet best suited to our highly individual nutritional needs? There are three major elements that you'll learn about in the following pages. For more detailed information, refer to my book, *Your Body Knows Best* (Pocket Books, 1996).

Metabolic Type

Your metabolic type is based upon your oxidation rate—the rate at which you turn your body's fuel, food, into energy. In the 1970s Dr. George Watson, a psychologist, identified two types of oxidizers: fast and slow. I refer to them as fast and slow burners. What these two categories of people have in common is that neither uses energy efficiently.

The slow burner doesn't process food quickly enough (due to underactive adrenals and thyroid), whereas it is speedily converted to energy in the fast burner (who has overactive adrenal and thyroid glands). The slow burner gravitates toward simple carbohydrates, sodas, and sugary foods for energy and tends to binge on starches. Generally, the appetite is poor and there is a dislike for protein-rich foods and fats.

The fast burner, on the other hand, will feel hyper, anxious, and irritable without sufficient fat and protein in the diet. A fast burner's appetite is generally strong, with a preference for heavy meats, and his emotional state is often characterized by peaks and valleys as energy levels fluctuate. While the slow burner tends toward poor circulation, low blood pressure, and dry skin, the fast burner is usually warm, perspires easily, and has high-normal to high blood pressure.

The slow burner does best on a diet emphasizing protein and, to a lesser extent, carbohydrates—although carbohydrates should not be consumed in excess. Protein can increase metabolism by 30 percent, while a pure carbohydrate meal increases it only 10 percent. Animal proteins of the lean variety (cod, tuna, eggs, and poultry) should be consumed as part of two meals each day. Purine-rich proteins, such as organ meats, are to be avoided and fat intake should be modest, as it will slow the metabolism further.

The fast burner will find a diet emphasizing fat and protein to be optimal. The heavier meats should be favored, and beef, lamb, venison, or cold-water fish should be eaten with every meal. These foods add substance and help balance out the highs and lows of the fast burner. Fats help slow down the overactive metabolism. Purine foods can be eaten freely. Both fast and slow burners should avoid processed carbohydrates such as bread, pasta, bagels, muffins, and crackers.

Not all people fall into these two categories. Some are normal or mid-range burners. They are generally able to maintain a desirable weight, due to their metabolic efficiency, whereas weight gain can be a problem for both the fast and slow burner. Eating in such a way as to restore metabolic balance helps to normalize weight and eliminate disease conditions.

These days, metabolic type can be determined through hair analysis. Questionnaires can also help a person determine his oxidation rate, as can increased awareness of the body and its response to food. The questionnaires beginning on this page will assist you in establishing your metabolic type and help in formulating a more personalized dietary plan. Answer "yes" or "no" to each of the following questions.

Slow-Burner Questionnaire	Yes	No
1. Are you somewhat laid back and even-tempered?	❑	❑
2. Does red meat feel heavy in your system?	❑	❑
3. Do you approach problems one step at a time, rather than juggling many things at once?	❑	❑
4. Can you skip breakfast without losing energy or getting hungry?	❑	❑
5. Do sweet things like candy or fruit give you a quick pick-up?	❑	❑
6. Do you prefer a "light" meal of salad and pasta rather than a "heavier" one of steak and potatoes?	❑	❑
7. Do you get thirsty often?	❑	❑
8. Do foods like cheese, butter, and avocados seem to make you feel sluggish?	❑	❑
9. Does coffee start your morning off just right?	❑	❑
10. Do you feel you need a pick-up from spices? Do you particularly enjoy tangy condiments like mustard, ketchup, and salsa with your food?	❑	❑

Fast-Burner Questionnaire	Yes	No
1. Do you consider yourself high-strung? Do you feel hyperactive?	❑	❑

Fast-Burner Questionnaire (cont.)	Yes	No
2. Do you actually feel better eating a plate of chops rather than leaner meats like chicken?	❑	❑
3. Do you enjoy a hearty high-protein breakfast, such as eggs and bacon?	❑	❑
4. Do you reach for salty snacks like nuts or potato chips when you're stressed out?	❑	❑
5. Are avocado, cheesy sauces, and full-fat dairy products very satisfying to you?	❑	❑
6. Do you feel better eating full meals every two to three hours?	❑	❑
7. When you eat sweet foods like cakes and cookies, do you burn out quickly after a short energy burst?	❑	❑
8. Do you have a hearty appetite?	❑	❑
9. Does drinking coffee make you nervous?	❑	❑
10. Does a pat of butter on toast satisfy you more than jam?	❑	❑

If you answered "yes" to eight or more questions in the slow-burner questionnaire, you are a classic slow burner type. If you answered "yes" to eight or more questions in the fast-burner questionnaire, you are a classic fast burner type.

Fast burners will do best on the 40/30/30 eating plan, while slow burners may feel better if they increase carbohydrates just a bit and lower the fats. If you fall somewhere between these two types, your current diet is probably serving you well.

Ancestry

Though the diet of humankind has undergone radical changes over the last forty thousand years, genetically, we have changed very little in that time. The climate of the land has always been the prime determinant of the foods available in it, and, over time, our ancestors adapted to changes in their environment and the diet it dictated. Those adaptations were genetically encoded in our lineage and, therefore, ethnic and genetic conditions persist regardless of how much people move around. Studies have demonstrated that the best diet for an individual is that of his or her native culture. Someone of American Indian heritage does best on a Native American diet of beans, squash, cactus, or buffalo, even if he moves to Japan. Changing locations does not change our genetic/nutritional needs.

Basically, we can think of our ancestral heritage in very broad terms, as indigenous to either northern or southern climates. The northern regions encompass Scandinavia, Canada, and northern and eastern Europe. These cultures adapted to diets high in cold-water fish, red meat, and root vegetables. The diets of people living in the southern regions featured light meat, fish, tropical fruit, beans, legumes, and light, water-based vegetables, such as lettuce, tomatoes, peppers, and cucumbers.

Because of the "melting pot" nature of our culture, most Americans have a mixed genetic heritage. Therefore, the genetic blueprint of our nutritional needs may not be that easy to decipher.

Blood Type

As I discuss in greater detail in my book *Your Body Knows Best* (Pocket, 1996), different blood types are related to the movement of generations of people over the continents, and they appeared at different times in our evolutionary cycle. Type O is the oldest type on the planet, followed by type A, then type B, and, finally type AB. The oldest types (O and A) are the most common in our culture today, with 85 percent of Americans falling into one or the other of these two categories. The rarest type of blood, type AB, was the last to evolve. People with this blood type make up only 4 percent of our culture.

As blood types evolved, nutritional needs evolved along with them. For example, people with type O blood are adapted to a diet heavy in animal meat and fish, and don't do well with dairy products or excessive consumption of grains. People with this blood type tend to lead an active lifestyle. Those people with type A blood also don't handle dairy well, and shouldn't overdo grains. However, these people are best suited to a semi-vegetarian diet (lean meat, poultry several times a week), and should not subsist on a diet that includes too many heavy meats. People with the third blood type to evolve, type B, can handle a wide variety of foods, including those from both the type O and type A diets, and can include dairy in moderation. And, finally, people with type AB blood are the only people fully adapted to dairy products. These people may have some type A characteristics, in that they have less tolerance for meat and animal products.

From this information, we can see that certain blood types would have a difficult time on a diet low in animal protein, while others would do much better on that type of diet. While most people in our culture have adapted to eating meat to some degree, few are able to handle dairy, according to blood type. It should be added that there are two subtypes of A, one better adapted to eating meat than the other.

The information on blood type and diet is fascinating, and research is ongoing in this country, thanks to the work of Dr. Laura Powers of Bethesda, Maryland. Japan is the home of the world's foremost authority on blood types and personality, Toshitaka Nomi.

GETTING STARTED

Start with your metabolic type. Once you know whether you are a fast or slow burner, you can modify your diet based upon blood type and ancestral heritage. If you do not have all of the information, work with the information you have. Use the 40/30/30 eating plan as a point of departure, regardless of other factors, and modify your diet according to what you know about ancestry, metabolic type, and blood type.

To obtain the full benefits of the 40/30/30 formula, you will need to follow it at every meal and at snack time as well. This is not a difficult task once you grasp the "how to" of applying the concept. You will find meal planning guidelines to help you achieve this goal in Chapter 11. These guidelines give sample meals, as well as tips to help you make your own balanced food selections.

The appeal of the 40/30/30 plan is that it avoids extremes of too much or too little in terms of macronutrient percentages. Diets that are extreme are appropriate for some individuals, and for these people, high percentages of macronutrients may be the answer to their dietary needs. But *extreme* diets should only be *temporary* diets. In the long run, they may push the individual past the point of balance into imbalance. And for those who are already out of balance, an extreme diet will push them further out of balance. This can be very damaging.

The Standard American Diet is approximately a 51/37/12 formula—51 percent refined carbohydrates, 37 percent saturated and "bad" fats, and only 12 percent protein. The protein content is inadequate in relation to the overabundance of fat and carbohydrates. For good health, you need to bring this into balance and switch to quality foods.

The stabilization of blood sugar that results from proper macronutrient balance helps control hunger and allows you to function optimally on less food (and therefore fewer calories) than you would normally consume. The advantages for weight control are obvious. There is also the potential benefit of increased longevity; animal studies have repeatedly correlated reduced food intake with increased life span. When macronutrient consumption is balanced, reduced food intake does not correlate with hunger: Satiety is more readily achieved naturally.

LOSING FAT WITHOUT LOSING MUSCLE MASS

Men seem better able to handle a larger carbohydrate load than women, most likely because of they have greater muscle mass and fewer fat cells. However, the basic hormonal response to food is not gender-specific. Men are no less vulnerable to the problems resulting from carbohydrate overload. Some men will lose weight on a grain- or pasta-based dietary regimen—lots of weight. They often lose more weight than they need to—and with it, muscle mass—and they're constantly hungry because they don't metabolize the grain protein well, and don't absorb enough nutrients from the food they eat. These men often overeat, prompted by constant hunger. Yet, the more they eat grains, beans, and vegetables, the thinner they get.

A diet devoid of meat, eggs, and dairy will result in a serious shortage of protein and essential minerals. You will sense that you are missing something, and because you are in a state of diminished nutrition, you will crave sweets. Giving in to these cravings will cause you to put on fat. This same cycle can be caused by diets that include some meat but are deficient in good oils.

Over the years, nutrition authorities and writers like Robert Atkins, M.D., John Yudkin, M.D., William Dufty, and Cass Ingram, M.D., have warned that sugar and starches (carbohydrates) can sabotage weight loss and set the stage for the development of degenerative diseases. The high-carbohydrate craze has born witness to the wisdom of their warnings.

Following a balanced eating plan—appropriate to your biochemical individuality—will assist you in ridding the body of unwanted fat. I use the word "fat" instead of "weight" because the two do not necessarily correlate. In fact, muscle weighs two and a half times what fat weighs. One can lose inches and look trimmer while maintaining the same weight or even putting on pounds.

I strongly urge you to have your body fat measured before beginning the balanced eating plan, and then again after thirty to sixty days. This can be done by measuring skin-fold thickness on various parts of the body with calipers; through hydrostatic, or underwater, weighing; or through bioelectrical impedance, which measures the body's resistance to a low-frequency alternating current.

How much fat you lose depends upon four variables:

1. The amount and type of carbohydrates you consume.

2. Your present level of fitness.

3. The amount of calories you take in.

4. The amount of calories you expend.

Remember also that total calorie intake should decrease with the 40/30/30 eating plan as appetite decreases.

On the low-fat/high-carbohydrate diet, very little of the weight lost is fat, for the insulin response bars access to the body's fat depots. On the other hand, eating a diet of balanced nutrient composition, adequate in protein, spares glycogen stored in muscles and the liver, and enables the body to burn fat, rather than to store it. Protein triggers the release of glucagon and drives the metabolism. With inadequate amounts, the body is hampered in its fat-burning ability.

Arnold, a thirty-four-year-old fitness buff, came to see me complaining that he could not lose weight even though he was working out daily and following what he believed was a healthy diet. Arnold believed in carbohydrates. After doing an extensive dietary assessment it was obvious that he also believed in the "more is better" theory. Arnold's diet consisted of enormous amounts of carbohydrates—like dry cereal, bagels, pasta, potatoes, fat-free muffins, and pita bread—eaten morning, noon, night, and in-between. After I explained to him the value of the 40/30/30 formula for weight loss and peak performance, Arnold agreed to include lean protein like eggs, white fish, and skinless turkey at every meal, and to add some butter to his bread and flax oil to his baked potatoes. He also agreed to reduce his gargantuan portions of carbohydrates, and learned to choose his carbs from the lower end of the glycemic index. Within three weeks, Arnold was burning fat and losing inches.

George, a forty-two-year-old office manager, was also having difficulty losing weight when he came to see me. He too had been following the high-carbohydrate/low-fat diet, but did not often exercise. After initially losing some weight on this diet, he had begun to gain it back. He told me he felt lethargic and craved sugar constantly. He felt totally out of control when it came to his eating. His dietary assessment revealed a shortage of good protein and a total lack of good fats. George thought he was doing the wise thing by cutting back on meat and eggs and consuming margarine and the "no cholesterol" vegetable oils from his local grocery store. But his body was starving for protein and healthy fats that level blood sugar and help control sugar cravings. Once we added butter and olive oil back into his diet, upped his protein intake, and cut back on the carbs, George began to lose weight again. And now that he has more energy, he has started working out in the gym.

Men need a higher ratio of protein than that contained in the Standard American Diet. This increased protein need is due to a catabolic metabolism that is tilted toward tissue breakdown. During sex, men discharge large amounts of stored protein, carbohydrates, and minerals. Men also tend to lose weight with greater ease, because they operate at a higher metabolic rate to maintain a higher percentage of muscle mass.

THE BOTTOM LINE

The challenge for today's man is not one of losing weight through dieting, but is instead an effort to achieve good health with proper nutrition. As with any extreme diet, the high-carbohydrate craze that has taken over the United States does not provide optimal nutrition. Instead, it appears that the heavy intake of carbohydrates in the Standard American Diet causes more health problems than it remedies, including blood-sugar disorders such as hypoglycemia and diabetes, food sensitivities, and obesity—to name only a few. The best thing that any man can do, then, is to cut back on his carbohydrate intake, and increase his consumption of the right kinds of fats.

Evidence now points to several fats, falling under the categories of omega-3 and omega-6 fatty acids, that are essential in maintaining health and preventing degenerative diseases. In fact, it's believed that a number of disorders correlate with EFA deficiencies, including alcoholism, coronary artery disease, obesity, and rheumatoid arthritis. Individuals on extremely low-fat diets are prone to deficiencies of essential fatty acids, and are therefore more likely to develop these and other conditions. However, paying close attention to EFA intake, and including good sources of omega-6 and omega-3 fatty acids in your diet can prevent or alleviate these problems.

The real key to regaining health and maintaining ideal weight lies in hormonal balance, which can be achieved with the right dietary ratio of macronutrients—carbohydrate, fat, and protein. Recent evidence has shown that the 40/30/30 balance of macronutrients is ideal for losing weight without compromising muscle mass. And while it cannot be claimed that any one diet is right for everyone, the 40/30/30 plan, with individual modifications based on metabolic type, ancestry, and blood type, can help stabilize blood sugar, decrease appetite, and increase fat burning.

3.

Quality Counts

Eating right is not as easy as it used to be. This may come as a surprise to you, given the variety of foods available to us today and, ideally, our diets should supply all of the nutrients we need to meet our daily requirements. Ironically, the abundance of selections on supermarket shelves make it more difficult, rather than easier, to plan nutritious diets. Today, too many of us consume a high percentage of readily available prepackaged foods that have had the nutrients processed right out of them.

This chapter will give you a behind-the-scenes look at the many processes that our foods undergo, from planting to harvesting to packaging. You'll learn how refining strips grains of their valuable antioxidants and other vitamins and minerals; why "enriched" does not mean "nutritious"; which food additives to avoid to lower your risk of cancer and other diseases; and how hydrogenation contributes to the development of fatty acids that have been linked to the development of heart disease. Within the following pages, you'll also discover how restoring homeostasis in your body with optimal electrolyte balance can help enhance your health—and even save your life.

FOOD PROCESSING

Food processing procedures include refining, enriching, hydrogenating, preserving, and irradiating. None of these processes enhances the food nutritionally. In fact, foods are processed for the sole purpose of extending their shelf life. And, because these processes actually result in considerable *loss* of nutrients, diets that include too much of these foods supply the bare minimum of nutrients necessary for survival.

Among the most heavily processed of our foods today are oil and grain products—these include all kinds of salad oils, cooking oils, and shortenings, breads, pastas, and pastries—anything made with white sugar and/or white flour. So one of the most fundamentally important changes a single man can make in his shopping and eating habits is to buy only unrefined oil and grain products. Look for these in your local health food store or in the "special foods" section of your supermarket. Select oils labeled *unrefined* or *expeller pressed* and breads made with whole wheat flour. Many labels simply say "wheat flour," which is a deceptive name for white flour—which is, of course, made from wheat.

Now, let's take a closer look at what happens to our food between the time it's harvested and the time when it's put on the shelves of our local supermarkets.

Refined Grains and Oils

All grains are not created equal. Much of what's available today has been refined, meaning that the husks of the grain have been removed. It is in these outer husks that most of the nutrients are concentrated. The part of the wheat plant that is made into flour and then into bread and other baked goods is the seed or kernel. The wheat kernel (a whole grain) has four main parts: the germ, the endosperm, the bran, and the husk. Typically, in the production of flour, the husk, bran, and germ are removed, resulting in extensive loss of nutrients. Wheat bran serves as a protective coating around the wheat kernel that is nutrient-packed and high in fiber. The germ is the part of the kernel that grows into a wheat plant, so it is rich in nutrients to support the growth of a new plant. Thus, only the endosperm, composed mostly of starch and protein, is left after whole grains have been refined.

During World War I, the milling of grains was forbidden in Denmark due to economic cutbacks. The death rate fell 34 percent and the incidence of cancer, kidney disease, and diabetes dropped significantly. During World War II, when grains were only partially milled in England, much the same thing happened. The less we refine food, the more it supports our health.

Among the nutrients lost in the refining process are the B vitamins, a family or *complex* of vitamins that plays an important role in nourishing the nervous system. We need extra amounts of the entire B family when we're under stress, but refined products— even those enriched with a few of the B vitamins put back—can't meet this increased need. A diet that has too large a proportion of refined food cripples the body's ability to deal with stress, which is a fact of life for today's man.

Also lost in the refining process are many of the important antioxidant nutrients—vitamins A, C, and E, and the minerals selenium and zinc. Antioxidants seek out and neutralize *free radicals,* the unstable molecules that are believed to play a key role in aging and to be involved in the development of degenerative diseases such as cancer. Free-radical formation is often caused by environmental stresses, including pollution, oxidation, exposure to ultraviolet radiation, ingestion of rancid oils, and surgery. We all need antioxidant nutrients to protect our bodies against free-radical damage. Consuming a diet of refined foods creates deficiencies in these important protective nutrients and therefore increases vulnerability to degenerative diseases.

In addition to the antioxidants removed in the refining process, much of the fiber of the whole grains is also lost. Fiber is a complex carbohydrate needed to move food residue through the intestines and prevent constipation. And many of the vitally important trace minerals are processed out, as well. According to Henry A. Schroeder, M.D., who did extensive research on the trace minerals over twenty years ago, "most of the energy in the average American diet, which comes from white flour, white sugar and fat, is not supplied with the trace substances needed to utilize that energy efficiently and properly."[1] The refining of sugar removes 93 percent of the ash—the trace minerals needed to metabolize the sugar—with it. The milling of wheat into refined white flour and the refining of raw cane sugar into white sugar remove minerals in the percentages shown in Table 3.1.

Table 3.1. Percentages of Nutrients Lost in the Refining Process

	White Sugar	White Flour
Chromium	93 percent	40 percent
Cobalt	98 percent	89 percent
Copper	68 percent	83 percent
Magnesium	98 percent	98 percent
Manganese	89 percent	86 percent
Zinc	98 percent	78 percent

Additionally, white flour has lost the following minerals originally present in whole wheat: 60 percent of the calcium, 71 percent of the phosphorus, 77 percent of the potassium, 78 percent of the sodium, 76 percent of the iron, 48 percent of the molybdenum, and 75 percent of the selenium.

Iron is the only mineral that is later added back to food in the enriching process, which we will discuss shortly. But enriching foods with iron can cause more problems than it solves, because iron that is added to the grain is in the form of inorganic iron sulphate, which the body is unable to absorb properly. The absorption problem is compounded by the lack of other minerals in refined foods. As a consequence, this iron often ends up being deposited in the arteries and joints, leading to degenerative disorders such as heart disease and arthritis. For example, in Sweden, liver cancer rates tripled when they began fortifying their flour with iron.

While inorganic forms of iron are not well absorbed, there are some natural iron supplements available, such as iron peptonate, that are more readily utilized by the body. The *heme* form of iron found in meat, poultry, and fish is also well absorbed, making liquid liver extract a good supplemental source of iron for those who need it.

Iron deficiencies in men are rare, however, except possibly among those who have low thyroid function, and those who have lost blood, been ill, or engaged in endurance exercise. As a general rule, men should avoid taking supplemental iron and consuming foods enriched with it, for iron overload can create serious problems, including heart disease, arthritis, diabetes, and impotence. Also, excess iron is stored in the central nervous system, and high levels of the free form of this mineral have been found in the brains of people with Parkinson's disease. If you suspect that your iron levels are low, consult your physician and have laboratory tests performed before you begin taking supplemental iron. (Chapter 6 explains more about preventing and detecting iron overload.)

The refining process removes most of the eight vitamins present in whole wheat, yet only three—thiamin, riboflavin, and niacin—are replaced in the enriching process. So, in the end, refining removes over two dozen nutrients and replaces only four.

White "polished" rice is also a refined product. After processing, it retains only the following percentages of trace minerals originally present in the whole grain: 17 percent of the magnesium, 25 percent of the chromium, 73 percent of the manganese, 62 percent of the cobalt, 75 percent of the copper, and 25 percent of the zinc. Therefore, it would benefit you to choose brown rice over white for a more nutritious meal.

As you will remember, when the bran and germ from whole wheat are removed, nothing is left but the starchy part of the kernel known as the endosperm. It's in this starchy portion of the grain that the heavy metal cadmium is concentrated. Cadmium toxicity is strongly associated with high blood pressure, or hypertension. If enough zinc is present in the body, it help can defend against cadmium toxicity. Unfortunately, zinc is contained in the bran and germ portions of the grain, and is therefore discarded in the refining process. This means that when we eat refined grains, we are vulnerable to the ill effects of cadmium—particularly if our body stores of zinc are low. And in the absence of chromium and fiber, also removed in the refining process, the body has trouble processing the starch that remains. Pure starch stresses the pancreas and throws the blood sugar into turmoil. These problems are not encountered when whole grains, rather than refined products, are included in the diet.

Most of the oils consumed in the Standard American Diet are also highly refined. According to Schroeder, separating oil from corn results in a refined product with less than 1 percent of the magnesium and only 25 percent of the original zinc. Vitamin E, needed to help retard spoilage, is also removed, as is lecithin, a fat emulsifier. The fat-digesting enzyme, lipase, is destroyed by the heat used in processing, making the oil indigestible. Beta-carotene is also virtually destroyed by processing methods. And, perhaps worst of all, refining destroys much of the valuable omega-3 and omega-6 essential fatty acids, which we discussed in Chapter 2.

Be aware of how oils are processed, the ingredients they contain, and what has been removed. *Unrefined* and *expeller-pressed* oils are the best products to purchase, because the oil is extracted without heat. A hydraulic press is used to crush the nuts, seeds, grains, olives, or vegetables, and the oil is squeezed out by force of pressure.

Manly Minerals

Many of the most important minerals for men are largely discarded in the refining process. Some, like selenium, are even deficient in our soils to begin with. All men should make sure that they are getting enough of the following minerals.

Calcium: When we think of calcium, we generally think of its valuable role in maintaining strong, healthy bones. In fact, 99 percent of the body's calcium is stored in the bones and teeth. If a calcium-deficient diet is consumed over a long period of time, the bones may become porous and brittle due to osteoporosis. Hip fracture is a common sign of osteoporosis, and one-third of all hip fractures occur in men.

The remaining 1 percent of calcium, distributed throughout the bloodstream and in extracellular fluids, performs many essential functions, as well. Men who consume foods rich in calcium or take calcium supplements tend to have lower blood pressure, and experience none of the unpleasant side effects that can be encountered with antihypertensive drug treatment.

Food sources rich in calcium include dairy products, such as milk, cheese, and yogurt; leafy vegetables, including collard greens, turnip greens, mustard greens, and sea vegetables; and salmon and sardines, including the bones. The recommended dose is from 800 to 1,500 milligrams daily. Calcium citrate is a form of supplemental calcium that's well absorbed by the body.

Chromium: An estimated 3 million men are unknowingly walking around with some of the early signs of diabetes. Chromium is an essential mineral that helps the body regulate blood-sugar levels, thereby protecting against full-blown diabetes. It also promotes the loss of fat and an increase in lean muscle mass. Two tablets of brewer's yeast will supply a day's need (from 200 to 800 micrograms) of chromium. Other notable sources include brown rice, cheese, clams, corn oil, grapes, honey, meat, raisins, and whole grains.

Copper: Copper is a double-edged sword. On the one hand, copper is a true warrior in the defense against heart disease and irregular heart rhythm. Plus, copper is an essential component of superoxide dismustase (SOD), a powerful antioxidant that is manufactured by the body. Copper deficiency can cause elevated cholesterol levels and blood pressure, and may actually lead to problems maintaining a normal heart rhythm.

On the other hand, copper overload is a common problem these days due to adrenal depletion and the copper content of dental fillings and water pipes. Copper toxicity can be an underlying cause of panic attacks and yeast infections.

Food sources of copper include liver, soy products, regular tea, cocoa, nuts, peas, beans, whole grain cereals, raisins, and oysters. The recommended daily amount for healthy males is about 2 milligrams.

Magnesium: Men who work out on a regular basis will want to maintain healthy magnesium levels, because this mineral plays a critical role in energy production and muscle activity. Research shows that magnesium may also help protect against heart disease, which kills more than 350,000 men each year, and can lower high blood pressure and cholesterol levels. Magnesium acts as a natural tranquilizer and, in fact, deficiency can interfere with the transmission of nerve impulses, resulting in irritability and nervousness.

Magnesium is found in most foods. Rich sources of this mineral include dairy products, fish, meat, seafood, green leafy vegetables, nuts such as almonds, and seeds. The recommended daily intake ranges from 600 to 1,000 milligrams per day.

Selenium: Selenium is an important antioxidant that protects the body against the formation of free radicals. As such, it is a valuable weapon in the fight against cancers of the skin, lung, and stomach that, combined, kill more than 100,000 men each year. Selenium is known to act in concert with vitamin E to protect cells from free-radical damage.

Depending on the selenium content of the soil where the food is grown, selenium can be found in meat and grains. Especially good sources include brewer's yeast, broccoli, brown rice, dairy products, seafood, and whole grains. The suggested daily intake for selenium ranges from 100 to 400 micrograms.

Zinc: Zinc is the most crucial mineral because of its link to male potency, fertility, and sex drive. A man may lose some 420 micrograms of zinc through ejaculation so, clearly, the more sexually active the man, the more he needs this essential mineral. Low zinc levels have been linked to low semen volume and low levels of testosterone. The mineral is also in small amounts through sweat, resulting in decreased levels.

As a component of the antioxidant enzyme superoxide dismutase (SOD), zinc helps the body to combat free radicals. It also promotes immune-system health and wound healing, and can be helpful in treating benign prostate hypertrophy (BPH), which commonly affects men over fifty. (See Chapter 5 for a discussion of BPH.)

Zinc is found primarily in red meats, eggs, and seafood. The recommended intake is about 15 to 50 milligrams per day. Zinc picolinate is the form that is best utilized by the body.

Enriched Grains

Enriched foods are those to which nutrients have been added in an attempt to replace vitamins and minerals that were lost in the refining process. However, "enriched" does not necessarily equal "nutritious," because the nutrients are generally put back in their inorganic forms, which are not well utilized by the body.

Another problem with the enriching process is that some nutrients are added without the vitamin and mineral counterparts needed for their utilization. For example, iron is replaced in enriched foods, while copper, which is essential for iron absorption, is not added. Unabsorbed iron adds to the body's storehouses and can be especially problematic for men because, overall, they do not need additional iron in their diets. Ultimately, all nutrients work *synergistically*, meaning that some vitamins and minerals enhance the function of other vitamins and minerals, enabling them to work better within the body. When any one nutrient is removed from the whole food, the activity of those remaining is adversely affected. Enriched food provides only a small portion of the full spectrum of nutrients needed for optimal health, growth, and strength.

Nutrient deficiency predisposes both plants and humans to disease conditions. Crops become infested with insects and then are treated with chemical pesticides. We medicate our sick soils in much the same way as we medicate ourselves when our bodies are invaded with germs. In both instances, the problem may well be averted by providing the host with nutrient-dense food—for the plant that is natural fertilizer, such as rock dust, and for humans, it is food grown in soils supplemented with natural fertilizer, known as organic foods. Organic foods are those grown without the use of chemicals that, as a result, show minimal toxicity and provide superior nutrition. They are becoming increasingly popular. In 1994, there were three thousand more certified organic farmers in this country than there were in 1990.

There is great variation in the mineral content of vegetables grown in different locations and under different conditions. Variable soil quality makes for variable food quality. The Firman

Bear report, as shown in Table 3.2 below, originally issued through Rutgers University in 1948, shows just how great these variations can be.

Table 3.2. The Firman Bear Report
Variations in Mineral Content of Vegetables

	Calcium	Magnesium	Potassium	Sodium	Manganese	Iron	Copper
SNAP BEANS							
Highest	40.5	60	99.7	8.6	60	227	69
Lowest	15.5	14.8	29.1	0	2	10	3
CABBAGE							
Highest	60	43.6	148.3	20.4	13	94	48
Lowest	17.5	15.6	53.7	0.8	2	20	0.4
LETTUCE							
Highest	71	49.3	176.5	12.2	169	516	60
Lowest	6	13.1	53.7	0	1	9	3
TOMATOES							
Highest	23	59.2	148.3	6.5	68	1938	3
Lowest	4.5	4.5	58.8	0	0	0	0
SPINACH							
Highest	96	203.9	257.0	69.5	117	1584	32
Lowest	47.5	46.9	84.6	0.8	1	19	0.5

Millequivalents per hundred grams / Trace elements ppm

Since this report is almost fifty years old and mineral depletion of the soils has greatly increased in the intervening years, we can assume that today's figures would be even lower than those cited above. Take a close look at this chart. It should be great incentive to go organic.

Food Additives

The U.S. Food and Drug Administration has approved some 2,800 food additives. These include chemicals added to extend shelf life, enhance flavor and color, and stabilize, thicken, and emulsify our foods.

Preservatives such as benzoates, sulfites, nitrates, and nitrites retard food spoilage by checking the growth of microbes—bacteria, yeasts, and molds and other fungi. Of these preservatives, benzoates are used most frequently. Sulfites are found in beer, wine, and dried fruit. Both of these additives can cause allergic reactions in some people, so they should be avoided by allergy-prone individuals.

Sodium nitrate and nitrite protect against bacterial growth and preserve food color. They are widely used today in curing meat and smoking fish. Packaged meats containing sodium nitrite should be avoided because, in the stomach, nitrites combine with products of protein breakdown called amines to form carcinogens (cancer-causing agents) known as nitrosamines. Nitrogen from chemical fertilizers is a documented source of nitrates. Seepage into underground aquifers can contaminate drinking water supplies. Vegetables, too, can absorb nitrogen compounds from fertilizers, and these are passed on to humans when we eat the plants. Bacteria in the stomach then convert the nitrogen compounds to deadly nitrites. When nitrites enter the bloodstream, they react with hemoglobin to form methemoglobin. The resulting disease, methemoglobinemia, causes the victim to turn blue from lack of oxygen. Suffocation and death may result.

Benjamin Feingold, M.D., found that a large percentage of hyperactive children are unusually sensitive to preservatives and to artificial colors and flavors. He found a link between food additives and learning and behavioral disorders. Today, hyperactivity is better known as *attention deficit disorder* (ADD). ADD affects a number of adults, as well as children, and is commonly treated with counseling, behavior modification techniques, and drugs. Since drugs destroy nutrients, thereby deepening deficiency, they can aggravate the problem by increasing sensitivity to adverse effects of food additives.

In truth, many of these additives are dispensable. Artificial colors, for example, do not provide any benefit, but are used only to make food look attractive. Dietary restriction of food additives is certainly a safer and, most likely, a more effective approach, as demonstrated by the success of the Feingold diet. Choose whole foods whenever possible to avoid preservatives and other food additives.

Hydrogenated Oils

Despite their bad reputation, saturated fats, consumed in moderation and in balance with other dietary components, will not harm a healthy body. The harm comes from the altered, damaged fats consumed in the typical American diet. Over the last century, a 350-percent rise in the incidence of cardiovascular disease has paralleled the rise in both sugar and processed oil consumption, but has not correlated with cholesterol consumption, which has remained about the same.

The myth still persists that substituting margarine for butter is the "heart smart" thing to do. The reasoning is that, because margarine is made from unsaturated vegetable oil, it is healthier than butter, an animal fat that is more saturated with hydrogen. But many people don't realize that margarine is created from unsaturated oils through the hydrogenation process.

Hydrogenation was first developed in 1912 by a Frenchman who created it as a means of hardening soap. The process involves supersaturating oil with hydrogen at temperatures exceeding 400°F, using nickel as a catalyst. Hydrogenated corn, soybean, safflower, and canola oils are a much greater health risk than are naturally saturated fats such as butter. The harm caused by these oils is partly due to the hydrogenation process, which destroys nutrients, including those needed for a healthy heart—vitamins E and B_6, and minerals chromium and magnesium. But to make matters worse, unhealthy fats called *trans fatty acids* (TFAs) are formed during hydrogenation.

The trans fatty acid molecule is strictly man-made. It does not appear in nature, and so the body has difficulty metabolizing it. Because vegetable oils typically have low hydrogen levels, it takes a long time to thoroughly saturate them during hydrogenation. During this time, harmful trans fats are formed. On the other hand, tropical oils—palm, palm kernel, coconut, and cottonseed oils— start out with a high level of hydrogen saturation. Because it takes much less time for them to become hydrogenated, TFAs do not form in the process. These fats do not have to be eliminated from the diet if they are regulated by the inclusion of essential fatty acids. (See Chapter 2 for a detailed discussion of essential fatty acids.) In fact, research has shown that, in some countries, people with a high intake of tropical oils have a significantly lower risk of cardiovascular disease, hypertension, and cancer than those of us in the United States.

A special word should be said here about cottonseed oil. Because cotton is considered a "non-food" plant, it is sprayed with numerous herbicides, pesticides, and fungicides. Residues of these poisons can be found in the seeds and in the oil from the seeds. I recommend avoiding cottonseed oil altogether in the diet. Remember that it's important to read product labels, because partially hydrogenated cottonseed oil is one of the major ingredients in processed and packaged foods.

Trans fatty acids usually remain in the blood, where they tend to increase "bad" LDL cholesterol and decrease "good" HDL cholesterol. A study printed in the British medical journal, *The Lancet* (March 3, 1993), warns that a high intake of trans fats may increase the risk of coronary death by as much as 50 to 67 percent. Altered fats also block the pathways used by the essential fatty acids, leaving the body deficient even when these good fats are part of our diets. This can adversely affect cell function and depress the immune system.

No one knows for certain what level—if any—of trans fatty acids can be safely tolerated by the body, but many researchers feel that amounts in excess of 2 grams a day should be avoided. To get a sense of how easy it can be to exceed that limit, take a look at Table 3.3 on page 46.

Consuming as little as 3 to 4 grams of trans fatty acids each day can lead to a 30-percent increase in the risk of cardiovascular disease. Industry officials and the federal government claim that Americans take in 8 to 10 grams of TFAs daily. Dr. Mary Enig of Silver Springs, Maryland, thinks this is an underestimate. She believes that the average American consumes between 11 and 28 grams a day, which is approximately 20 percent of total daily fat intake.

Table 3.3. Trans Fatty Acid Content of Common Foods*

Food	Trans Fatty Acid Content
Chocolate chip cookies	11.54 g
Processed American cheese	8.07 g
Danish pastry (one large)	6.63 g
Sugared donut	5.28 g
Apple turnover	5.23 g
Crackers made with partially hydrogenated soybean oil (10 small)	4.36 g
Margarine (1 Tbsp.)	3.50 g
Vegetable shortening (1 Tbsp.)	2.70 g
Butter (1 Tbsp.)	0.50 g

* From *Trans Fatty Acids in the Food Supply: A Comprehensive Report covering 60 Years of Research* (Enig Associates, Inc., 1993) by Mary G. Enig, Ph.D.

To avoid TFAs, you'll need to eliminate vegetable shortenings, margarine, processed cheeses, commercial baked goods, mayonnaise, candy bars, processed peanut butters, and microwave popcorn from your diet. Make a habit of reading labels and avoiding anything that says "hydrogenated" or "partially hydrogenated."

MAINTAINING ELECTROLYTE BALANCE

Electrolytes are mineral salts that conduct electrical energy when dissolved in solution. In the body, the bloodstream provides the fluid medium for electrolytes to carry out this function. Electrolyte deficiency or imbalance results in energy loss, leaving us feeling fatigued—a common complaint. No wonder, considering the scarcity of vital trace minerals necessary for electrolyte formation in the body. As we've already discussed, deficiencies are widespread today, owing to the depletion of our soils and depletion through food processing—so we won't find our food supply to be a reliable source of trace minerals.

Fatigue is the first symptom of just about everything. When we have insufficient energy to run the body, its processes break down

Mars Bars, Minute Rice, and Margarine: A Flawed Study

In doing the research for this book, I ran across a scientific study that stopped me dead in my tracks. It focused on the effects of carbohydrates and fats on energy levels in the human body. What was appalling about it was that the carbohydrates used were in the form of Minute Rice and Mars Bars, and the fat used was margarine. All of these are highly processed foods, altered from their natural states. The resulting nutrient loss makes them fragmented foods that react very differently in the body than do natural, whole foods. Processed foods are unbalanced in their nutrient composition and therefore create imbalances in the body, disrupting normal physiological processes and leading to disease conditions. To draw conclusions about how the body responds to carbohydrates and fats in general based on how it responds to these unnatural, devitalized ones in particular is not accurate and can give rise to the formulation of erroneous data.

The potential benefits of the 40/30/30 formula cannot be achieved if you eat a diet made up of 40 percent refined carbohydrates, 30 percent hydrogenated fats, and 30 percent protein from animals who "do drugs." The benefits of the three major nutrients, carbohydrates, fat, and protein, are seriously compromised when vitamin and mineral content is altered, as it is in today's foods. That's why quality counts.

and we feel tired and sluggish as a result. Adequate levels of electrolytes, then, are crucial to our health. Without enough of these vital elements, we can't maintain *homeostasis*, our body's balancing mechanism. When electrolyte balance is disrupted at any level, energy flow is disturbed and chemical processes that are needed for good health are adversely affected, leading to development of disease conditions. As Henry A. Schroeder, M.D., tells us in *The Trace Elements and Man* (Devin-Adair, 1973), homeostatic mechanisms will break down under two conditions: 1) a deficiency of vital trace elements, and 2) an excess of vital elements.

Cultures that enjoy exceptional health and longevity drink mineral water that cascades down from mountain streams and swirls over rocks, creating vortexes. This whirling motion generates an electrical charge in the minerals taken up by the water, changing them from a colloidal to a much more bioavailable, or readily absorbed, crystalloid form. In this manner, nature creates electrolytes, which are fully assimilated by the body, owing to their crystalloid form.

Two of the most effective ways of purifying water are the distillation and reverse-osmosis methods, both of which remove minerals in addition to pollutants. If you use these methods, then you're going to need to add trace minerals back to the water. However, most liquid mineral formulas on the market are colloidal in nature. *Colloidal minerals* are inorganic elements that cannot fully penetrate cell walls, and are not well utilized by the body. Additionally, many come from sources that are contaminated with heavy metals.

We can duplicate nature's electrolyte formation by adding crystalloid minerals back to our purified water. A liquid mineral supplement containing the correct minerals in the correct amounts and in a crystalloid form constitutes a true electrolyte formula. The only such formula available on the market today, to the best of my knowledge, is a product called Trace-Lyte.* Regular use of this product will help restore electrolyte balance.

Restoring electrolyte balance assists the body in combatting virtually any disorder by eliminating conditions that gave rise to it. Among those basic conditions is pH imbalance, which can be corrected through the regular use of Trace-Lyte in combination with a balanced diet. A balanced diet alone cannot be counted on to regulate pH, however, in the face of electrolyte imbalance. This is unfortunate because pH balance is one of the body's major defenses against disease. Another is *osmotic equilibrium*, the equalization of force or pressure between the inside and outside of cell walls. The restoration of osmotic equilibrium strengthens cells and makes them unfit hosts for bacteria and other germs. This restoration is accomplished by re-establishing homeostasis through electrolyte balance. Electrolytes must be in balance for certain beneficial bacte-

---

* Trace-Lyte is available through Uni-Key (1–800–888–4353).

ria to exist and carry out their function of fighting harmful bacteria. Therefore, the proper functioning of the immune system depends upon electrolyte balance.

Many scientific papers written in the last twenty years indicate that by restoring pH and osmotic equilibrium, we may significantly decrease our risk of infection. In addition to normalizing pH and osmotic pressure, electrolytes have also been proven to help restore peristaltic action of the bowel muscles; increase digestive efficiency; increase oxygen to the cells; reduce water retention problems; correct neuromuscular imbalances; improve enzyme production; regulate blood-sugar levels; increase energy levels; and strengthen the immune system.

Trace-Lyte can be used as an electrolyte supplement, and it can also be used to remineralize purified or distilled water. Just add one teaspoon to each gallon of water. Taken in conjunction with other nutritional supplements, it will enhance the activity of electrolytes by improving assimilation. If very large amounts of isolated minerals are taken over a long period of time, however, we run the risk of disrupting balance once again, since excessive mineral intake as well as deficiency can cause a breakdown of homeostatic mechanisms.

While inorganic forms of minerals may form deposits in various organs and tissues of the body—causing such problems as kidney and gall stones, hardening of the arteries, constipation, and arthritis—the crystalloid form will not do so. In fact, it will actually help eliminate existing deposits by creating balanced conditions that allow the minerals to go back into solution. Crystalloid minerals, as electrolytes, likewise play an active role in "escorting" heavy metals out of the body. They are nature's own chelators.

Overabundance of some minerals can create deficiencies of others. Ideally, we want to incorporate mineral-rich whole foods, such as sea vegetables, into our diet, as a highly usable and balanced source of organic minerals. Sea vegetables include nori, dulse, hijiki, wakame, arame, kombu, and agar-agar. These are good in vegetable soups and natural gelatins.

A FINAL WORD

In order to choose quality macronutrients, it's necessary to become educated about what "good quality" means. Quality foods include fruits and vegetables grown organically, meat obtained from organically raised animals, "fertile" eggs laid by chickens that roam free, sea vegetables, whole grains, and unrefined oils. Quality beverages include fresh fruit and vegetable juices, herbal teas, and purified water to which electrolytes have been added.

Packaged, canned, and bottled items should be avoided as much as possible. Never purchase these items without first checking the label, even in a health food store. Avoid artificially sweetened foods and all products containing hydrogenated or partially hydrogenated oils, as well as commercially processed dairy products, packaged meats, and smoked fish. Shop the outside aisles of your supermarket—where the whole foods are—and patronize your local health food store.

Remember that, although the nutrients you need for good health are not always available in the foods you buy, you can compensate for nutrient loss from soil depletion and food processing by choosing organically grown whole foods and taking nutritional supplements. In addition, the regular use of a true electrolyte formula can help you restore balance, or homeostasis, to the body. This will assist in the prevention of disease conditions and aid in recovery from all types of illnesses.

4.

Protein
Makes a Comeback

Lean protein—the white meat of poultry, flank steak, eggs, and fish—is a cornerstone of super nutrition. It can make the difference between optimum nutrition and malnutrition. Protein, which comes from a Greek word meaning "first," is appropriately named because it is the most important of the macronutrients, found in virtually every cell of the body. Eating enough of the right kind of protein can transform your body into a fat-burning machine and give you extended energy, improved concentration, and appetite control.

Back in the 1970s, we were advised to eat as much protein as possible. Nutritionist Adelle Davis had us counting protein grams instead of calories. By the 1980s, however, we were loading up on carbohydrates in preference to proteins, wary of cholesterol problems we were taught would result from eating high-protein meat and dairy products.

The pendulum has swung one way, then another, and has finally landed in the middle—the point of balance. As we have come to recognize the hormonal effects of food, the merits of protein are being examined in a new light. However, rather than a "more is better" approach, we're seeing the importance of balancing protein intake with carbohydrate and fat. We are learning that by increasing protein intake in relationship to carbohydrates, we trigger a favorable hormonal response.

As you will remember from Chapter 2, protein activates the fat-mobilization hormone, glucagon, which assists us in losing weight, building lean muscle mass, stabilizing energy levels, controlling hunger, and so forth. When the 40/30/30 balance is achieved, appetite is normalized. Consequently, so is caloric intake, which diminishes as hormonal balance is established. This is not a high-protein diet, for the actual amount of protein consumed daily according to the 40/30/30 eating plan might remain the same as it was before—or even decrease. Many men can adjust the ratio simply by reducing their carbohydrate intake.

Because it boosts metabolic rate, increased protein intake can be especially beneficial to the slow burner, giving him more energy and better endurance. Increasing metabolism can help burn off stored fat and improve utilization of energy from foods.

PROTEIN BASICS

Next to water, protein is the most plentiful substance in the body, comprising 50 percent of our body's weight. Proteins are made up of building blocks called *amino acids*—twenty-three of them. When you eat protein-rich foods, your body breaks the protein down into its amino acid components, and then uses these building blocks to manufacture new proteins. Thousands of proteins are made from different combinations of these twenty-three amino acids. Some are used by the cells to build new tissue, others to construct antibodies, hormones, enzymes, and blood cells.

Of the twenty-three amino acids, eight are considered *essential*, meaning that they can't be produced by the body, but must be supplied in the diet. These are isoleucine, leucine, lysine, methionine, phenylalanine, threonine, tryptophan, and valine. Two more amino acids, arginine and histidine, are essential in the growth period of life and sometimes, due to acquired or genetic factors, in adult life as well.

Protein controls the catabolic/anabolic cycle of the body. In the catabolic phase of this cycle, muscle tissue is broken down during strenuous physical activity, whereas it is built up in the anabolic phase. Increasing protein intake in the diet facilitates the formation of new muscle. Muscles contain more protein than any other structure of the body. Men need more of it—and more calories—because of greater muscle mass and because their metabolism leans toward the catabolic. In addition to these functions, adequate protein is needed for:

- Blood clotting
- Building new cells
- Energy production and endurance
- Formation of hormones
- Formation of the brain's neurotransmitters
- Healthy hair, skin, and nails
- Maintaining strong immunity
- Muscular strength and tone
- Normal digestion
- Regulation of fluid balance
- Stimulation of metabolism
- Tissue growth and repair

A food is considered a *complete* protein if it contains all of the eight essential amino acids. Complete proteins include meat, fish, poultry, milk, and dairy products. Bee pollen and spirulina also fall into this category. Of the meats, liver and kidney have the highest protein value in terms of their amino-acid profiles.

DIETARY GUIDELINES

It's recommended that men take in about 50 to 75 grams of protein per day. Of course, individual needs vary, based upon nutritional status, body size, and activity level, as well as genetic factors. For example, athletes (especially bodybuilders) need more protein than less active men. To stimulate muscle growth, weight lifters should take in approximately 1 to $1^1/_2$ grams of complete protein per pound of lean body weight, while endurance athletes require $^2/_3$ to $^3/_4$ grams of protein per pound of lean body weight.

High-protein meal replacement formulas are frequently used for weight loss and supplemental protein. Those containing casein should be avoided. Casein is a difficult-to-digest milk protein to which many men are allergic. Commercially, it's used to glue wood together because of its tenacious adhesive quality. The casein content of cow's milk is 300 times higher than mother's milk and a by-product of its bacterial decomposition is mucous production, yet another strike despite the fact that it is a complete protein. Meat is a better choice for complete protein—meat from free-range chickens, wild game, and antibiotic- and hormone-free beef.*

Eggs are also an excellent source of complete protein. They are one of the few food sources of the sulfur-containing amino acid, L-cysteine, which is essential for healthy skin, hair, and nails. Their cholesterol content should not be a concern, for high dietary cholesterol does not translate into high cholesterol in the body. Another bonus is that eggs have a high lecithin content. As a fat emulsifier, lecithin is a cholesterol-lowering agent. One can safely eat eggs every day, though powdered eggs should be avoided. The cholesterol in powdered eggs is oxidized and therefore toxic to blood vessels.

Since soybeans are a complete protein, the vegetarian would do well to make liberal use of tempeh and soybean products such as tofu in his diet. He should make sure, however, to supplement zinc to offset high copper levels in all soy products. Soy's health benefits give the meat-eater a reason to incorporate it into his diet as well. The entire soybean family of plant chemicals provide protection against cancer, and any of the foods made from soy significantly lowers blood cholesterol and reduces the risk of heart disease.

Other excellent plant protein sources include honeybee pollen and sesame seeds. Bee pollen contains all of the essential and nonessential amino acids. Its therapeutic effects include regulation of metabolism and oxygenation of cells. Many athletes and Olympic stars have found bee pollen to be very beneficial. As a supplement, 1 to 2 teaspoons can be taken daily with food or bev-

* A company called Lean and Free (1–800–383–BEEF) raises hormone and antibiotic-free cattle. Their beef can be ordered by mail and shipped throughout the country. Other companies that provide organic beef include: Country B3R Meats (Childress, Texas) and Coleman Natural Beef (Denver, Colorado). Organically raised chicken and turkeys from Shelton Farms, Harmony Farms, Foster Farms, and Young's Farms are sold through health food stores and cooperative buying clubs.

erage. When starting supplementation, it is best to begin by taking a smaller amount (try half a teaspoon) and to increase gradually.

Another fine vegetarian source of complete protein is the blue-green algae spirulina. Along with bee pollen, spirulina is considered to be one of the world's most perfect foods. It's a rich source of natural protein (60 to 71 percent) that is more digestible than most foods because it lacks cellulose, a plant fiber that cannot be digested by humans. It is also rich in vitamins, minerals, and EFAs.

It has been estimated that the average man's protein consumption represents only 12 to 18 percent of total daily calories. Therefore, for most men, the challenge is not so much one of adding more protein grams, as it is balancing protein intake with carbohydrates and fats—and, of course, upgrading the quality of all macronutrients. There are problems associated with both underconsumption and overconsumption of protein.

Food Combining

It has traditionally been taught that in order to properly synthesize protein, the body must be supplied with all essential amino acids simultaneously in the proper proportions. For example, plant foods do not contain sufficient amounts of all of the essential amino acids. They are, therefore, said to be *incomplete* proteins. Grains lack lysine and threonine, while beans lack methionine. By combining grains with beans at the same meal, the amino acid profile is complete.

This practice, however, is not in vogue anymore. Current teaching dictates that complementary proteins can be eaten during the course of the day rather than at the same meal. I am personally in favor of the current teaching for another reason: Eating grains and beans together can create an overload of carbohydrate, leading to excessive insulin production and its fat-promoting properties in sensitive individuals.

AVOID EXTREMES

I've already stressed the importance of maintaining a healthy balance and avoiding dietary extremes, such as high-carbohydrate diets. Moderation should be extended to your intake of protein, as well. Since both excess and deficiency of protein can cause problems, the heavy meat-eater and the vegetarian alike can be in trouble. Vegetarians often develop problems that stem from deficiency, while heavy meat eaters may suffer from conditions related to toxicity.

Protein Deficiency

Protein deficiency may lead to abnormalities in growth and tissue development. The protein-deficient man often has poor posture because he lacks the muscle tone and energy to stand perfectly erect. He may also have a diminished sex drive, constant food cravings, thinning hair, and brittle nails. The mental state is often characterized by irritability, depression, and confusion. A study of Massachusetts Institute of Technology students found that protein significantly improved their ability to do mental tasks, while carbohydrates curbed this ability by making them more relaxed. This is most likely because proteins produce dopamine and norepinephrine, two chemicals in the brain that boost alertness.

The protein-deficient man may also be bloated and overweight due to insufficient *albumin*, a blood protein that makes urine collection possible. Inadequate protein can't support albumin formation and water leaks out from the cells into the spaces between them where it can't be excreted by the kidneys.

Insufficient protein can result in poor resistance to infection, impaired wound healing, and delayed recovery from illness. Antibodies are the body's chemical "bullets" for the fight against pathogens such as viruses and bacteria. An antibody is, by definition, a blood protein. Without enough dietary protein, antibodies can't form and immunity is impaired. Also made of protein are phagocytes, or "killer cells," a form of white blood cell important to our immunity. So, too, are enzymes. Protein deficiency thus creates an inability to produce adequate quantities of enzymes. This adversely affects digestion, which in turn hampers the body in its ability to utilize other nutrients.

The deficiencies that can occur in a vegetarian diet are numerous, especially if the diet is vegan (devoid of eggs and dairy, as well as flesh products). Plasma and urine tests conducted at Aatron Medical Services reveal that vegetarians are commonly deficient in the amino acids lysine, methionine, tryptophan, carnitine, and taurine. The first three of these are essential amino acids. Lacking these, the body can develop immune and liver dysfunction, weight problems, and sleep disorders.

Because vitamin B_{12} is found only in animal products, vitamin-B_{12} deficiency is common among vegetarians. Pernicious anemia is the classic sign of B_{12} deficiency, but other symptoms can include dementia, depression, paleness, and numbness and tingling in the extremities. Vegans should consider supplementing with 500 micrograms of vitamin B_{12}.

Less well known is the fact that vegetarians are often zinc deficient. This mineral is critical for proper immune and reproductive functions, and for maintaining stable blood-sugar levels. The typical vegetarian diet is high in copper. This can give rise to such conditions as skin problems, yeast infections, lowered immunity, depression, lack of mental focus, and, in extreme cases, schizophrenia.

> *Roger, a twenty-five-year-old graduate student had begun eating a vegetarian diet after reading a very popular diet book in the late 1980s that touted food combining and vegetarianism. For several years he felt marvelous. He had more energy and more mental clarity. Then slowly but surely, his energy levels reached a plateau and began to slip. He also began to experience recurring colds and bouts of flu.*
>
> *After reviewing his high-carb, low-protein diet history, I immediately added fish and chicken to his eating program on a daily basis. Roger also agreed to include at least four eggs a week in his diet. His energy picked up almost immediately. And his bouts with colds and flu have subsided to one cold or so a year.*

Protein is used to build new cells to replace those that are constantly lost from day to day, such as skin and hair cells. Stresses, such as injury, surgery, hemorrhage, and prolonged illness cause a loss of body protein. Supplemental protein may therefore be indicated at times of stress; however, excessive protein intake may cause fluid imbalance and other problems.

When Is Vegetarianism Appropriate?

In consideration of metabolic type, ancestry, and blood type, I believe it's fair to say that a vegetarian diet is not appropriate for the majority of men. A man with type-O blood who is a slow burner of Northern European heritage cannot maintain health on a vegetarian or even a semi-vegetarian diet. However, he may find, as other types have, that such a meatless diet is effective as a short-term therapeutic regimen, particularly if it incorporates plenty of fresh vegetable juices. Vegetables contain a number of unique substances that possess healing properties, including carotenes, flavonoids, and chlorophyll, as well as thousands of phytochemicals. But most important, vegetables—especially vegetable juices—provide high levels of minerals needed by the body to form electrolytes and reestablish homeostasis.

Since all other nutrients, including protein, require minerals for their activity, saturating the body with minerals from fresh vegetable juices (and, ideally, taking Trace-Lyte) in times of illness becomes a priority. Because juices provide no fiber, however, it's also necessary to consume fiber-rich whole vegetables, as well. Fiber helps to detoxify and build up the body. Once the body is built up to the point where digestion is normal, due to restoration of pH balance provided by the electrolytes and the alkaline ash of the vegetables, extra protein is needed to build new tissue and complete the healing process. Providing high-protein foods prematurely, however, simply adds to the body's toxic burden. Without the digestive ability to break the protein down into its amino acid components, the protein will putrefy and thus postpone recovery, rather than assist it.

If high-protein foods of animal origin are not added back to the diet of the recovering man at the appropriate time, when his metabolic rate, blood type, and/or ancestry dictate a need for it, he will deteriorate. Because of these factors, some men will do better on a maintenance diet of lean meats eaten more frequently; others will fare better on lighter proteins like fish and foul eaten less often. Most men should avoid dairy. I feel confident in saying that all men should incorporate some animal products into their diets— even just a few eggs a week. Diets of healthy peoples around the world have traditionally been composed of highly nourishing foods and devoid of junk food and empty calories, but they have all included some animal products. This was confirmed by Dr. Weston Price (himself a vegetarian) in his classic study of the diets of indigenous cultures in the early 1900s.

The healthy man may benefit from incorporating fresh vegetable juices into his diet on a routine basis and may even wish to use them exclusively for a day or two to cleanse his system and help replenish his alkaline minerals reserve. Such a mono-food diet, however, should not be extended beyond a few days because of the inherent lack of macronutrient balance.

Protein Toxicity

Seventy-two percent of the protein consumed by Americans comes from animal products. Consuming excessive amounts of meat in the absence of fiber-rich carbohydrates will cause constipation and putrefaction of protein with resulting toxicity. A high intake of animal protein has been linked to osteoporosis and kidney stones. The link found here is in the effect of excess protein on calcium metabolism. When protein intake is increased from 47 to 142 grams daily, the excretion of calcium in the urine doubles.[1] Alkaline minerals (primarily sodium and calcium) are needed to buffer the acid ash left from consumption of meat. Usable forms of these minerals are obtained primarily from fruits and vegetables, which are sparse in the Standard American Diet. According to Senate Document #436, published in 1936, 99 percent of Americans are mineral deficient!

Overconsumption of acid-forming foods, such as meat, forces the body to rob its own storehouses—taking sodium from the muscles and calcium from the bones and teeth—to provide alkaline minerals to neutralize the acid caused by excess protein consumption.

> *Paul and Mike were twenty-something weight-lifters who wanted to get real "mean and lean." They each began following an extremely high-protein diet, consuming 8-ounce steaks twice a day. They believed that combining this with their weight-lifting would stimulate fat burning and build muscle mass. In a little less than a month on this overdose of protein, both came to see me on the recommendation of a friend. Paul had suffered a stress fracture in his right wrist, and Mike complained about his whole body feeling tight and his lower back constantly aching.*
>
> *It appeared that both these men were forcing their bodies to rob their bones for calcium and their muscles for sodium. I immediately switched them to the 40/30/30 plan and put them on Trace-Lyte Electrolytes. I also advised both of them to choose fat-free cottage cheese to help replenish calcium and sodium reserves. Within eight days both reported feeling better, with a leveling of mood swings, and relief of lower back pain.*

A high intake of animal protein has also been linked to heart disease, high blood pressure, and kidney disease. While excessive intake of saturated fats contained in animal products can be a risk factor in the development of coronary-artery disease, lack of EFAs, overconsumption of sugar, and macronutrient imbalance are perhaps more important, though less recognized, factors. A word about cholesterol: Cattle of today store a different kind of fat in their muscles than did the animals of the past. These animals were range-fed on grasslands, but today they're fed grains and injected with the growth hormone, stilbestrol. Whereas the grass-fed cattle accumulated a fatty acid called oleic acid in their muscles, today's beef cattle store a different kind of fat, called stearic acid, which contributes to the elevation of "bad" low-density lipoprotein (LDL) cholesterol.

THE TRACE MINERAL CONNECTION

Most people assimilate only a small percentage of the protein they take in, generally about 20 percent. Most people are also deficient in trace minerals needed for electrolyte formation. There is a relationship between the two previous statements. Read them again. Trace minerals enable the body to use proteins. By returning the needed minerals to our soils and our bodies, electrolyte balance would be reestablished. We would assimilate a greater percentage of the protein we eat and therefore need less of it. In the face of trace-mineral deficiency, homeostasis is disrupted due to electrolyte imbalance, body pH is thrown off, and digestion is impaired, limiting our ability to produce enzymes to break down protein and other nutrients. According to Gillian Martlew, N.D., author of *Electrolytes: The Spark of Life*:

> *Filling up with protein or large amounts of separate amino acids unaccompanied by electrolytes saturates the body with harmful waste products. This is caused by the incomplete conversion of protein to amino acids. In this situation, the body creates uric acid instead of new tissue, and is then forced to use more minerals trying to neutralize it. . . . The enzymes needed for digestion are created from amino acids with the help of electrolytes. Minerals enable proteins to be broken down into their component parts (amino acids), which then become bioavailable—available for body use.*[2]

Protein, then, is essentially useless and toxic to the body in the absence of electrolytes needed to produce the enzymes necessary to break it down into amino acids. It is highly recommended that all men include supplemental trace minerals in the form of a true electrolyte formula (containing liquid minerals in crystalloid form) in their diet on a regular basis.

POINTS TO PONDER

Throughout the decades, we have been urged to include large amounts of protein in our diets, and then to cut back on protein in favor of carbohydrates. Fortunately, in recent years scientists and nutritionists have begun to appreciate the beneficial aspects of protein when it's consumed in proper balance with carbohydrates and fats. Increased protein intake boosts metabolic rate and activates glucagon, the body's primary fat-mobilization hormone.

For a protein to be considered complete, it must contain all of the twenty-three essential and nonessential amino acids—the building blocks of proteins. While meats and dairy products are well known as good sources of complete proteins, there are many foods not derived from animals that can supply all of the necessary amino acids. These include soybeans, sesame seeds, and spirulina, a type of blue-green algae, and they are all excellent sources of protein for the vegetarian male who does not take in protein from animal products. A full range of essential and nonessential amino acids can also be consumed through food combining, in which complementary proteins are eaten during the course of the day to complete the amino acid profile.

As you strive to balance your intake of protein with carbohydrate and fat, remember that protein is basically useless in—and even toxic to—the body without enough of the minerals that are essential to protein assimilation. These minerals, in the form of electrolytes, produce the enzymes that are needed to break down protein into its constituent amino acids, which are then made available to help run and repair the body. So it's a good idea to include supplemental trace minerals in your dietary regimen.

5.

Protecting Your Prostate

The prostate gland is about the size of a walnut and is located at the base of the bladder, surrounding both the urethra and the ejaculatory duct. This duct connects into the urethra and opens up into it. The prostate acts as a valve that permits both sperm and urine to flow in the proper direction. It is an accessory sex gland that assists in the reproductive process by secreting an ejaculatory fluid that enhances the delivery and fertility of sperm. Secretion from the prostate gland constitutes about 80 percent of the fluid volume of semen. The prostate receives sperm from the testicles, produces nutrients that nourish it, and assists in the passage of that sperm. It also serves to protect the genitourinary system against infection.

Prostate problems stem from genetic, hormonal, and dietary factors. While you may have no control over your genes, you do have control over your diet, which directly affects hormonal factors. When it comes to problems with the prostate, choosing "watchful waiting" and proper nutrition over aggressive medical treatments may be the best medicine of all. We've already seen some of the ways in which hormonal output can be influenced by food. Prostate problems, brought on by a lifetime of bad eating, can be turned around by dietary changes that support the gland by re-establishing hormonal balance.

Adequate intake of essential fatty acids, which you learned about in Chapter 2, is absolutely critical for the good health of the prostate. By increasing the right fats in your diet, from nuts, seeds, and supplemental oils, you can significantly support and nourish your prostate gland, decreasing your chances of developing any of the problems outlined in this chapter. The best initial medicine may be the essential fats, and avoidance of the nonessential, harmful trans fats from margarine, vegetable shortenings, fried foods, and processed vegetable oils. (For more information on trans fats, refer to Chapter 3.)

The increase in trans-fat consumption over the past several decades can be correlated with a dramatic increase in prostate disorders. Harvard researchers Walter Willett and associates suggest there is a positive correlation between dietary intake of the trans fats and the rise of cancer. And it seems that the culprit is not as much animal fats as vegetable fats, because statistics show that the consumption of animal fats has decreased by 30 percent since the beginning of the century, while vegetable-fat consumption is up 30 percent. In addition, you've been told time and again that men whose diets are high in saturated fat—particularly red meat—run the greatest risk of developing prostate cancer. Well, that's just part of the story, because what's missing from this advice is recognition of the critical role of the EFAs in balancing and regulating saturated fats.

This chapter begins with a look at the most common prostate problem faced by today's man—benign prostatic hyperplasia. We'll then go on to discuss several other conditions that you should be aware of, including prostatitis and prostate cancer. You'll also learn about a variety of natural and nutritional supplements that can help to keep your prostate gland healthy.

BENIGN PROSTATIC HYPERPLASIA

During childhood, the prostate gland is quite small—just a little larger than a pencil eraser. Its growth and functioning are controlled by the male hormone *testosterone*, which at puberty facilitates not only prostate growth, but growth of sex organs and body hair, as well as change of voice. By the time a man reaches age twenty, his prostate gland has achieved full size. However, after age forty it begins to enlarge. This growth is hormone induced.

While testosterone levels have begun to decline by this stage of life, production of one of its metabolites, dihydrotestosterone (DHT), increases. The enzyme that converts testosterone to DHT is testosterone 5-alpha reductase. DHT levels increase within prostate cells as a result of increased activity of this enzyme, as well as a greater uptake of testosterone and a lower rate of breakdown and excretion of DHT. This increase is associated not only with prostate enlargement, but also with male pattern baldness, because 5-alpha reductase is partly concentrated in the scalp. The enzyme is also found in scrotal skin and in the testicles. It appears that the aging process brings on both the decline of testosterone production and the increased conversion of testosterone to DHT. An increase in this conversion is what gives rise to growth of tissue in the prostate gland.

Benign prostatic hyperplasia (BPH) is the nonmalignant enlargement of the prostate gland that primarily affects men over fifty. The incidence of the disorder increases with age. By age fifty, approximately 30 percent of all males in this country will begin to experience the symptoms of BPH. By age sixty, half will be affected. Beyond the age of seventy, almost 80 percent of all males will develop the disorder. And, by age eighty, almost every man in the United States will have BPH. It is the main problem treated by urologists. Some consider it to be a natural consequence of aging.

Prostate enlargement results in urethral constriction and the development of BPH symptoms, including weak stream of urine, dribbling, progressive frequency, urgency, hesitancy, and intermittence of urination. It's a condition that can be painful. Men with prostate enlargement often have to get up three to five times a night to urinate. In 2 to 3 percent of BPH cases, urinary incontinence results from instability of the outer muscle layer of the bladder, known as the detrusor muscle. Any man experiencing these symptoms is strongly urged to consult a physician for a definitive diagnosis. If left untreated, the condition can result in complete blockage of the bladder outlet, causing uremia, or urine retention in the blood.

Benign prostatic hyperplasia can lead to cancer. An estimated 20 percent of those with BPH will develop prostate cancer. While prostate cancer was relatively rare before 1900, it is increasingly prevalent today. Like BPH, it is most common in later years. Only 2 percent of all prostate cancers occur in men under fifty. (Testicular cancer, on the other hand, is most common in the younger age groups, primarily affecting those men between fifteen and thirty-four years of age.) In 1994 alone, 200,000 cases of prostate cancer were diagnosed, with thirty-eight deaths resulting from it.

Conventional Treatments

Surgery is the most commonly recommended treatment for BPH. There are three different surgical procedures, but *transurethral resection of the prostate* (TURP) is the surgery performed on 95 percent of all patients. Four hundred thousand of these procedures are done each year. In fact, it's the most common surgery performed on men over sixty-five.

TURP involves removal of the central core of the gland to take pressure off the urethra. A significant complication in this surgery is excessive absorption of irrigating fluid that causes what is known as TURP syndrome, characterized by nausea, vomiting, and mental confusion. Left untreated, TURP syndrome can lead to high blood pressure, heart failure, and seizures.[1] The surgery claims a 90-percent success rate. However, according to Dr. John Weinberg of Dartmouth Medical School, the death rate has been as high as 1.8 percent (one death per fifty-six procedures), 8 percent are hospitalized within three months because of complications, 5 percent (one out of twenty) become impotent, and about 20 percent (one out of five) will need another resection.[2]

In addition to TURP syndrome, complications from this surgery include temporary and, more rarely, permanent incontinence and retrograde ejaculation, in which the man ejaculates backwards into the bladder instead of into the penis. Retrograde ejaculation affects one-half or more of TURP patients.

The drug considered to be most effective in controlling BPH symptoms acts by blocking the conversion of testosterone to DHT. The drug finasteride (Proscar) does this by inhibiting the enzyme testosterone 5-alpha reductase. Proscar has been on the market for only about three years. It works slowly, taking approximately three months to accomplish maximum shrinkage (about 28 percent). It must be taken indefinitely and, like most drugs, Proscar has undesirable side effects. These can include impotence and decreased libido. The medication is also costly—several dollars per day. Even so, annual sales are expected to top $1 billion dollars this year. The cost of hospital care and surgery for BPH in the United States is also over $1 billion dollars per year. Fortunately, a less expensive, less invasive, safer, and more effective approach to BPH management may be found in nature's pharmacy.

Saw Palmetto Extract

Saw palmetto (*Serenoa repens*) is a small palm tree that grows along the Atlantic coast from South Carolina to Florida. An extract from its berries has proved to be an effective remedy for prostate enlargement. This herb has been used for centuries by herbalists and Native Americans to treat urinary tract problems, and has also been considered by some to be a mild aphrodisiac.

The French pioneered research in the clinical use of saw palmetto for BPH, establishing that its mode of action is the same as Proscar—that is, it blocks the formation of DHT by inhibiting testosterone 5-alpha reductase. It has also been found to display other modes of action that prevent DHT uptake by the prostate cells and therefore is described by French scientists as a multi-site inhibitor.

One double-blind study involving 110 men with benign prostatic hyperplasia found after one month that the group using the herbal extract improved as follows: decreased nighttime urination (nocturia) of more than 45 percent; increased urinary flow rate over 50 percent; and reduced amount of urine retained in the bladder following urination (post-urination residual volume) by 42 percent. In contrast, the placebo group showed only slight reduction in nocturia, no improvement in urine flow, and increased post-urinary residual volume. Ratings of outcome by physicians and patients both showed "significant" improvement in the group treated with saw palmetto. This was not so for the placebo group.[3]

European research indicates that the greatest therapeutic benefits of saw palmetto are found in the fat and sterol portions of the plant. This finding has given rise to the production of a standardized extract of the fat-soluble, or liposterolic, fraction of saw palmetto berries. There are many types of preparations on the market and some are more potent than others, as Table 5.1 indicates.

Table 5.1. Potencies of Available Saw Palmetto Preparations

Type of Saw Palmetto	Relative Strength to 85–95% Extract
Dried berry	5%
Liquid tincture extract	5–10%
Powdered extract (4:1)	25%
Liquid oil extract (10:1)	50%
85–95% Liquid oil extract (20:1)	100%

It is the last item, the liquid oil 20:1, that is used in the European clinical studies. It contains 85 to 95 percent sterols and fatty acids and, in the studies, was given in amounts averaging 320 milligrams per day. The program I have developed (see Appendix B) includes the most potent extract of saw palmetto.

Treating prostate disease with saw palmetto extract has not only been proven to be extremely effective, but it costs less than a third as much as prescription remedies, and it is safer. Between 1983 and 1992, nine double-blind studies conducted involving 528 benign prostatic hyperplasia patients have concluded that the extract of saw palmetto was effective. This conclusion was based upon both objective and subjective measurements of prostate enlargement. And all studies demonstrated no toxicity.

In addition to saw palmetto, natural progesterone cream for men may beneficial in preventing prostate enlargement. Dr. David Zava, a noted progesterone researcher, will be reporting on the use of natural progesterone in the treatment of both prostate enlargement and prostate cancer in his forthcoming book. Uni-Key Health Systems (1–800–888–4353) now carries the product Progesta Care for Men.

Nutritional and Herbal Support

Inadequate diet appears to be a primary factor in the development of BPH. For this reason, the condition usually responds to nutritional and herbal support, especially in the early stages. The extent of dietary advice that most doctors are likely to dispense is apt to be limited to the recommendation that spices, alcohol, caffeine, and other irritating foods be avoided and that the fluid intake be kept high. This is good advice, but there's more to it.

Perhaps the most important element in a nutritional program to prevent or treat BPH is the trace mineral zinc. Zinc deficiency is common today because the soils of thirty-two states are deficient in the mineral. It is also removed in processing and is depleted by smoking, alcohol, coffee, infections, and medications. The ability to absorb zinc declines with age. A normal prostate gland contains more zinc than any other organ in the body. Because the prostate serves as a zinc storehouse, some believe that when zinc is needed elsewhere, the body robs the prostate, thus depriving it of this critically important trace element.

Zinc (as well as vitamin B_6) plays an important role in many aspects of hormonal metabolism. This may be why it's effective in reducing prostate size and symptoms of prostate enlargement. Good sources of zinc include brewer's yeast, eggs, meat, organ meats, seafood (especially oysters), seeds, and soybeans. Vitamin B_6 also plays an important role in nourishing the prostate gland.

Other nutrients important to prostate health include vitamins C and E and the mineral selenium. These are all antioxidant nutrients, needed to offset free radical-damage to cells and preserve oxygen, that are generally deficient in the SAD. Two other powerful antioxidants used for prostate problems are Pycnogenol from pine bark and grape-seed extract. These extracts are rich a source of substances called anthocyanidins and proanthocyanidins, both pigments known as flavonoids that have exceptionally powerful antioxidant effects.

Extra amounts of the B complex vitamins will help the body to deal with the stress of any illness, including benign prostatic hyperplasia. Stress increases the need for this family of vitamins. And an increased intake of vitamin A will help prevent and/or resolve infection. Beta-carotene, a precursor of vitamin A, can be used as well.

Adding nuts and seeds to your diet, or increasing your current intake, is a tasty way to provide an extra source of both zinc and the essential fatty acids. A deficiency of these "good" fats seems to be a major factor in the development of BPH. So, increasing the intake of EFA-rich oils from various nuts, as well as flaxseed and evening primrose oils, has a regulating effect on the saturated animal fats in the diet. It's not simply a matter of decreasing animal fat and protein, as has been generally recommended, but one of balancing total fat intake with good fat.

Prostatic and seminal lipid (fat) levels and ratios are often abnormal in people with BPH, and significant improvement can be attained by administering an EFA complex containing linoleic and linolenic acids.[4] It would appear that a prostaglandin deficiency may be a cause of BPH. Since EFAs are precursors to prostaglandins, they are vital to normal prostate function.

Pumpkin seeds are a rich source of both EFAs and zinc, so the folklore medicine remedy of eating $1/4$ to $1/2$ cup of these seeds daily for prostate problems may indeed have value. Pumpkin seed oil, found in most health food stores, may also be used. In addition, remember that a high-carbohydrate diet should be avoided and all forms of sugar (including fruit, fruit juice, and sweeteners) should also be severely limited, because they stress the hormonal and immune systems.

If you suffer from BPH, you may also benefit from taking a glandular extract, or protomorphogen, of prostate tissue. These are produced from bovine (cow) and porcine (pig) sources. Raw glandular concentrates appear to provide the pattern from which the body can build new cells. Healthy bovine or porcine prostate extract ingested by a man with prostate enlargement is more beneficial, it seems, than actually eating the organ meat itself. After being refined, raw glandular tissue assumes an enzymelike action that improves assimilation by the target organ—in this case the prostate.

It has been found that exposure to cadmium from cigarette smoke, paints, contaminated drinking water, and shellfish found near industrial shores will stimulate the growth of human prostatic tissue, and that proper concentrations of the mineral selenium will inhibit that growth.[5] Those men with BPH will want to rule out cadmium toxicity. This can be done through hair analysis.

Amino acids can also be used to treat BPH. One study indicates that supplementation with a combination of L-glutamic acid, lalanine, and glycine (two 6-grain caps taken three times daily for two weeks, followed by one cap taken three times daily) may be beneficial. The study, involving forty-five patients supplemented with this combination of amino acids, showed reduction or relief of nocturia in 95 percent of the cases, urgency reduced in 81 percent, frequency reduced in 73 percent, and delayed urination in 70 percent.[6]

Another factor to consider is lactobacillus deficiency in the body. Low levels of these "friendly" bacteria can result in prostate trouble, hair loss, and abnormal fat distribution. Supplements of acidophilus bacteria can therefore be helpful. Bear in mind, however, that these beneficial bacteria will not grow in the intestines unless the body pH is near perfect, and pH is regulated by our old friends, the electrolytes. So you'll want to add these trace minerals to your supplemental regimen.

In addition to saw palmetto, the powdered bark of the *Pygeum africanus* tree has been useful in the treatment of benign prostatic hyperplasia. It has been used for centuries as a treatment for urinary disorders, and has also been found by French scientists to have anti-inflammatory properties and no toxic side-effects—even in large doses and with prolonged use. Clinical trials have proven its efficacy in alleviating symptoms. Another herb useful in this

regard is *Aletriusfarnosa* (star grass). And stinging nettle is also recommended by herbalists for BPH.

PROSTATITIS

Prostatitis, which involves inflammation or infection of the prostate gland, is most common in men under fifty. The infectious
variety can be either acute or chronic and is caused by a pathogen
such as a bacteria or chlamydia, which is a sexually transmitted
parasite. When there is a deficiency of glandular elements such as
zinc, vitamin C, and proteolytic enzymes that break down proteins, favorable conditions are established for infection to develop.
The glandular elements can be depleted as a result of excessive
consumption of caffeine, alcohol, and spicy foods, which leads to
lowered immunity. Increased sexual activity can lead to the development of prostatitis, for it depletes the prostate gland of enzymes
and zinc, nutrients that sterilize the urethra and protect the gland
from infection.

Symptoms of acute prostatitis include difficulty urinating characterized by frequency, urgency, and a burning sensation during
urination, as well as a discharge from the penis following bowel
movements. Prostatic pain and tenderness, which can extend into
the pelvis and back, are sometimes present at the outset of an acute
infection, and may be followed by fever, chills, and generalized
fatigue.

Symptoms of chronic infection are similar, but not as severe.
Because these symptoms are somewhat mild, some men may
ignore them. This is not wise because, left untreated, a chronic
infection of the prostate can result in infection in the kidney or the
tube along the back of the testicles known as the epididymis, as
well as swollen, painful testicles (orchitis), bladder outlet obstruction, and prostate stones.

Nonbacterial prostatitis is the most common form of this condition. The symptoms are the same as for bacterial prostatitis, but
no infectious agent is located, though white cells are present in
prostatic fluid, a sign of inflammation. The cause of this condition
is unknown. Both acute and chronic prostatitis are commonly

treated with antibiotics—short-term for acute and long-term for chronic. The nonbacterial type may also be treated with prostate massage, hot baths, antispasmodics, tranquilizers, and anti-inflammatory medication.

Another type of prostatitis, known as prostatodynia, involves essentially the same symptoms as described above, but no abnormalities are found on examination or through urinalysis. This condition is thought to be due to muscle spasms and is generally treated with medication and hot baths.

Herbal Treatments

Herbal preparations may be useful in the treatment of prostatitis. An evergreen plant known as pipsissewa (*Chimaphilia umbellata*) is useful for chronic infectious prostatitis, as well as other urinary disorders. It contains a powerful antiseptic, arbutin, which helps nourish the urinary tract and prostate and increase blood flow to them. Arbutin is also the active ingredient in uva ursi, a diuretic herb that is beneficial to the urinary tract.

Horsetail, a rich source of the trace element silica, may be useful in the treatment of acute prostatic infection. An herb that assists in fighting any type of infection, including prostatitis, is *Echinacea angustifolia.* Garlic also has natural antibiotic properties. Other herbs that may be useful for decreasing pain, irritation, swelling, and impotence associated with prostatitis include: *Delphinia staphysagria, Thuja occidentalis,* and *Anemone pulsatilla.* These herbs are frequently administered in homeopathic form. Homeopathy is a system of healing based on the use of very small amounts of substances, which in larger doses would cause illness in a healthy person, to treat illness. A homeopathic remedy is prepared through the dilution and potentiation of a small amount of the herb that becomes energized through the process.

Supplementation with vitamins, minerals, and essential fatty acids as outlined for benign prostatic hyperplasia is recommended, emphasizing increased intake of vitamins A and C where infection is present. Extra amounts of calcium and magnesium can help relax muscles.

PROSTATE CANCER

Prostate cancer is known as a "silent" cancer because few symptoms are usually felt initially. As the tumor grows it tends to constrict the urethra and present the same symptoms as BPH. It has been noted that BPH can lead to prostate cancer and that its onset generally occurs in the later years of life. In fact, the average age at diagnosis is seventy-three years old. One out of every eight men will develop prostate cancer in his lifetime.

The prostate is one of four sites in the body that accounts for more than half of all cancer deaths. The other three are lungs, colon, and breast. While breast cancer is infrequent in men, lung cancer is the number-one killer, prostate cancer is number two, and colon and rectum cancer run a close third.

Because its onset is usually late in life and because it is most often a slow-growing cancer, it has been argued that watchful waiting should take preference over aggressive treatment. Many men die of other causes before prostate cancer creates any real problem, and medical treatment, including surgery and radiation, can produce complications such as loss of bladder control, impotence, and rectal injury. According to autopsies, over half of all men over the age of fifty have cancerous prostate cells, but only 2.4 percent eventually die of the disease. Many men with prostate cancer, unaware of its existence, die of an unrelated cause. The cancer isn't discovered until an autopsy reveals its presence.

For these reasons, some view early detection of this cancer as a questionable benefit. There are no studies showing that early screening for prostate cancer can actually save lives, and the death rate for the cancer has remained pretty much unchanged for decades, despite advances in medicine. Techniques used for diagnosis include digital rectal exam (DRE), blood tests, tissue biopsy, and a number of visualization techniques such as x-ray, MRI, ultrasound, and CT scan that provide an image of the structures inside the body.

In the DRE, the physician will perform a rectal exam, feeling the prostate through the wall of the rectum. Hardness indicates a possible cancer, though it may also be due to infection or stones.

The DRE may be normal even when cancer is present, though this is unlikely. The American Cancer Society recommends annual DRE examination for all men over forty.

A common blood test for diagnosing cancer is the prostate-specific antigen (PSA) test. This test was developed in 1989. In its first year of use, it increased the number of diagnosed cases of prostate cancer by 16 percent. Even before that, diagnosis—and subsequently treatment—was increasing. From 1984 to 1990, surgical removal of cancerous prostates in men sixty-five and over increased 500 to 600 percent.

The PSA test is used to detect or confirm both BPH and cancer. Prostate-specific antigen is a protein substance unique to the prostate. It is slightly elevated in cases of BPH and greatly increased in men with prostate cancer. Infection can also cause elevation of PSA levels. The higher the PSA level, the greater the chance of metastasis, meaning that the cancer has spread to other parts of the body. When prostate cancer spreads, three-quarters of the time it spreads to bone. Some men do not seek medical attention until they experience symptoms of widespread disease, including fatigue, weight loss, and bone pain.

Nutritional advocate Julian Whitaker, M.D., voiced concern in the November 1994 edition of his newsletter, *Health and Healing*, that the increasing use of PSA screening will lead to increased use of surgery, radiation, and chemotherapy—and they have. These treatments have the potential of doing harm. He points to a study done in the *Journal of the American Medical Association*, which concluded that neither early detection, nor conventional treatment of prostate cancer resulted in a significant extension of life span. They did, in fact, reduce the quality of the patient's remaining years, due to side effects such as impotency.

Dr. Whitaker states that, in his own practice, he uses the PSA test in a different way—as a barometer of the success of nutritional treatment that includes saw palmetto and dietary changes. The power of conservative nutritional regimens is reflected in dropping PSA levels, witnessed many times by Dr. Whitaker.

I personally would suggest that more physicians take the Whitaker approach. I encourage all of my male patients in their early forties and fifties to start supplementing with saw palmetto as soon as possible, and banish trans fats from their lives forever.

You see, PSA results are not as clear-cut as one would hope. In 1993 it was reported that approximately 40 percent of men with prostate cancer show up negative; of those having no symptoms, but a positive PSA, only one out of 75 to 150 actually do have cancer, and false positives occur in one out of four men with symptoms. These statistics refer to the standard PSA test. A new PSA test has recently been developed that is said to be more reliable. A problem with false positives is that the suspicious results will generally prompt a biopsy, which carries with it some risk; therefore, it is desirable to reduce the number of low yield prostate biopsies being performed. Steps are being taken in this direction and a sixteen-year study designed to resolve the controversy as to whether early screening, detection, and treatment actually does extend the lives of men with prostate cancer is now underway.

Now there is a less invasive medical approach to treating early-stage prostate cancer. It involves a relatively new procedure in which radioactive pellets are implanted into the prostate gland. This procedure is done on an outpatient basis; it is therefore less costly than surgery and results in more rapid recovery and in fewer complications. One study, which involved 298 prostate cancer patients, found that 91 percent of those receiving the treatment were free of cancer five years later, compared with 82 to 89 percent of those treated surgically.

The American Cancer Society recommends annual PSA tests for all men fifty and over. They also recommend that high-risk men be tested annually beginning at age forty. High-risk men include African-Americans and men with a family history of prostate cancer. Based on new studies, we can add men who have had vasectomies to the list. The problem with vasectomies is that sperm builds up in the sealed-off vas deferens and is reabsorbed by the body, which reacts by launching an autoimmune response to its own tissue.

African-American men have the highest incidence of prostate cancer in the world. Their risk of developing it is 40 percent greater than it is for white American men. The interesting thing is that, while African Americans have a death rate from prostate cancer that is almost double that of white American men, the incidence of the cancer in black Nigerian men is only one-sixth that of black Americans. Another interesting fact is that, while prostate cancer death rate in Japan is only one-seventh of ours, when Japanese men relocate to America, their cancer rate rapidly increases.

The Dietary Connection

These statistics point to a cultural factor influencing the development of prostate cancer—one that overrides genetic influences. That factor involves lifestyle and diet. Our men typically lead a stressful, fast-paced life, are exposed to environmental toxins, and regularly consume a diet of devitalized, processed junk food. Please remember that prostate cancer was relatively rare before 1900—that is, before the advent of food processing, the widespread use of pesticides and other environmental toxins, and the fat-free, high-carbohydrate diet.

A major difference in diet with regard to the above referenced cultures is this: The Japanese and Nigerians eat much less animal fat and many more vegetables than we do. Numerous studies have indicated that the nutrients and *anutrients*—fiber, pigments, and phytochemicals—in vegetables have a protective effect against cancer and, of course, we've all heard of the link between heavy meat consumption and cancer. A 1993 Harvard School of Public Health Study found that men who eat red meat five times a week are 2.6 times more likely to develop advanced, often fatal, prostate cancer than are men who eat red meat one time or less weekly.[7] The balanced use of essential fats in the diet would probably change this situation dramatically.

Though a source of saturated fat, meat in and of itself is not a bad food. Meat from organically raised animals can be an excellent source of vitally needed protein, eaten by a healthy man with an adequate intake of EFAs, fiber, vitamins, minerals, and other nutrients. However, a man with cancer is not healthy. For him, excessive consumption of meat—especially without the addition of omega-3

EFAs from such oils as fish and flaxseed—will create conditions of further imbalance. Being out of balance, his body lacks the trace minerals to form electrolytes that must be present to produce enzymes necessary for breakdown of protein into amino acids. Additionally, the hydrochloric acid needed for protein digestion declines with age and will, most likely, be inadequate in the middle-aged or older man with prostate cancer.

Supplements of HCl and proteolytic enzymes can be helpful to support the digestive process until it can be normalized by the restoration of electrolyte balance through the regular use of Trace-Lyte in combination with a balanced diet.

Environmental Risk Factors

There is an established link between pesticide use and cancer. Our crops are treated with 1.2 billion pounds of pesticides and herbicides yearly. Studies have shown that farmers run a higher risk of developing certain cancers, including cancer of the prostate.[8] Over 600 pesticides are currently used in the United States. The Environmental Protection Agency has identified sixty-four of them as potentially cancer-causing. The EPA sets tolerance levels for pesticides in raw and unprocessed foods. The FDA is responsible for enforcing the levels set by the EPA. However, they do not test for all pesticides and actually screen only a very small percentage of our food supply—probably less than one percent. In addition, foods that are found to exceed the legal limits of pesticide residues are not prevented from going to market!

Imported produce has perhaps twice the level of pesticide residue that domestic food has, and should therefore be avoided. Pesticides banned in this country are often exported to other countries that use them on their crops and then import them back to us! In addition to washing or soaking produce to remove pesticide residues, it is wise to assure a high intake of fiber, chiefly from vegetables, and antioxidants—such as vitamins A, C, and E, and the minerals selenium and zinc—in the diet to help eliminate pesticides from the body.

In addition to avoiding pesticide residues in food, you will also want to avoid environmental exposure to chemicals. Instead of using chemical pesticides to rid your home of roaches and fleas, use natural alternatives or call in a natural pest control service. And use organic fertilizers on your lawn, rather than chemical ones.

The man with prostate cancer will, of course, want to avoid smoking and avoid exposure to secondhand smoke, as well. Cigarette smoke is a major source of cadmium toxicity. Studies show that cadmium may promote cancer by replacing zinc in the prostate.[9]

Exposure to electromagnetic fields (EMFs) appears to be another factor in the development of prostate cancer. Studies show that EMFs can suppress the pineal gland's secretion of the hormone melatonin. It is the suppression of this function that has been implicated in the etiology of prostate cancer. Melatonin plays a key role in preventing and reversing cancer. It increases the cytotoxicity of the body's natural killer lymphocytes, thereby inhibiting tumor growth. Clearly, it's important to limit exposure to EMFs as much as possible by keeping electrical appliance use in your home to a minimum.*

Another environmental factor that affects the likelihood of developing cancer has to do with exposure to sunlight. If you're thinking that such exposure increases the risk, you've got it backwards. The sun converts cholesterol in our skin to vitamin D, a vitamin that Duke University researchers have found to be protective against prostate cancer. A University of North Carolina study showed that men living in the northern latitudes, with less exposure to the ultraviolet rays of the sun are at greater risk for developing prostate cancer.

John Ott has done a great deal of research on the beneficial effects of sunlight. To reap its benefits, we must take in the rays—all of them, including UV—through the retina of our eyes. Spending at least half an hour outside, even in the shade, without glasses or sunglasses to block UV rays, can therefore be an important part of a prevention or recovery program.

---

* For further information on the detrimental effects of EMFs and how to avoid or reduce them, contact the Baubiologie Institute at (813–461–4371).

Preventing and Treating Prostate Cancer

Since prostate cancer symptoms are, for the most part, identical to BPH symptoms, all of the nutritional advice given for BPH applies to prostate cancer as well. Since those with BPH may later develop prostate cancer, they may want to incorporate some of the nutritional advice given in this chapter for that condition. While zinc levels are low in BPH patients, they're even lower in those with prostate cancer. So, zinc supplementation becomes especially important for males with prostate cancer.

Nutritional and herbal therapies can help prevent and treat prostate problems. Avoidance of sugar, damaged fats, processed foods, and the use of key elements such as antioxidant nutrients and especially the mineral zinc and herbs such as saw palmetto and the food spice, cumin, can be particularly beneficial. Outlined in the next few pages are several other simple measures you can take to keep prostate problems at bay.

Eat Your Vegetables

Italian and Swiss researchers compared 8,077 people with nineteen different types of cancer with 6,147 people without cancer. The individuals were placed in one of three possible groups: those who ate less than seven vegetables per week, those who ate seven per week, and those who ate more than seven per week. They found that a man who eats seven servings of vegetables per week has 20 percent less risk of developing prostate cancer than one who eats fewer than seven. And, a man who eats more than seven servings has a 70-percent less chance than one who eats less than seven. Seven vegetables per week is only one per day, and yet, even that small amount confers some protection. We should at least triple that amount.

The National Cancer Institute recommends that Americans consume a minimum of three to five servings of vegetables daily. Most Americans, especially men, fall quite short of this, even though a serving is only half a cup. Vegetables provide a wide range of nutrients and anutrients. They are not only a source of vitamins and minerals, but also of carbohydrates and protein. Among plant pigments are carotenes, flavonoids, and chlorophyll. Beta-carotene is just one of over 400 carotenes. All have potent antioxidant and anticancer effects. One large, ten-year study involving 2,440 men, ages fifty and older, showed an inverse relationship between serum vitamin A and prostate cancer incidence. The men who developed the cancer had significantly lower vitamin A levels than those who did not develop it.[10]

Tissue-carotene content can be increased by juicing a wide variety of vegetables, a practice highly recommended for cancer patients. The nutrients in freshly prepared juices are concentrated and are easily used by the body. Flavonoids provide protection from free-radical damage. They are found largely in fruits and flowers. Pycnogenol and grape-seed extract are part of this group. They are extremely potent antioxidants. The green plant pigment chlorophyll has also been shown to have significant antioxidant and anticancer effects.

Vegetables are best consumed in their fresh state. Use frozen in preference to canned if fresh is not available, and select organic whenever possible. If commercially grown vegetables are used, wash or soak them first in a 3-percent hydrogen peroxide solution (preferably food grade) to remove pesticides, molds, and bacteria. A diluted Clorox solution may also be used, but only with purified water, as the pollutants in water will unite with chlorine to form potentially carcinogenic compounds. Using the Clorox bath has the added benefit of killing parasites (a growing health hazard discussed in Chapter 8). To prepare a Clorox bath, add a half teaspoon of bleach to a gallon of purified or distilled water. Soak the food for fifteen to thirty minutes, then soak in clear water for ten minutes.

Vegetables should not be overcooked, as this destroys important nutrients. The best cooking methods are light steaming, baking, or quick stir-frying. Never boil vegetables, unless they're being made into soup.

One vegetable in particular, the Japanese maitake mushroom, has shown promise in treating prostate and other types of cancer. Naturopathic physician Peter D'Adamo, editor of the *Journal of Naturopathic Medicine*, has reported success in his private practice in Greenwich, Connecticut, using maitake to treat men with prostate cancer in whom chemotherapy has been unsuccessful. The mushroom has also been used with success by Dr. D'Adamo in treating pulmonary metastasis, in which the cancer has spread through the lungs and circulatory system, and cancers of the liver, breast, and colon. Others have reported that maitake helps combat chronic fatigue syndrome, high blood pressure, diabetes, and human immunodeficiency virus (HIV), the virus that causes AIDS.

Abraham Ber, M.D., a homeopathic physician who practices orthomolecular medicine in Phoenix, Arizona, also reports success with using the maitake mushroom in his practice over a two-year period. He has treated at least a dozen prostate cancer patients with maitake tablets and obtained encouraging results, including improved urinary flow and decreased frequency.

These mushrooms have a powerful strengthening effect on the immune system. Maitake is considered to be an *adaptogen.* It assists the body in adapting to any form of stress and helps regulate endocrine activity and other body functions to achieve balance, or homeostasis. It has recently been found that maitake mushrooms taken by patients undergoing standard chemotherapy reduced the amount of chemotherapy drugs needed by 50 percent without compromising the anticancer results of the treatment.

Recent findings, based on a study conducted at Memorial Sloan-Kettering Cancer Center in New York, indicate that men who regularly consumed the common spice cumin had a significantly lower rate of urological cancers, including prostate cancer, than those who consumed little of the spice.

Joe was a fifty-five-year-old contractor who sought my services after being diagnosed with prostate cancer. He had decided not to go the "traditional" route with chemotherapy and wanted to discuss the watchful waiting approach. After reviewing his chart and assessing his dietary history, we drew up a dietary regimen with herbal support.

My first recommendation was to eliminate all trans fats from his diet. Joe's love affair with McDonald's French fries was over. I strongly advised that he cut back on his meat consumption and only use sources that were organic. Increasing his zinc and essential-fatty-acid intake was accomplished with the addition of nuts and seeds—specifically pumpkin seeds—to his diet. I also recommended that he supplement with evening primrose and flax oils, as well as additional zinc. Supplemental saw palmetto and antioxidant nutrients, including Pycnogenol, vitamin C, vitamin E, and the mineral selenium were included in his treatment plan as well as maitake mushroom extract. Joe felt strongly that a nutritional regimen was his best bet, and he could always resort to chemotherapy if he needed it. So far, so good.

Enhance Your Immunity With Natural Supplements

When you use herbs for prostate cancer, keep in mind that they are not specific for the different types of tumors, but act rather as overall immune system stimulants. In addition to the herbs mentioned in the BPH section, the following can help treat prostate cancer: poke weed, mistletoe, meadow saffron, foxglove, poison hemlock, and burdock.

Other immune-enhancing herbs that may be useful include: pau d'arco, ginseng, licorice root, and goldenseal. Additionally, coenzyme Q_{10} and Royal jelly will assist in building immunity and strength in both men with prostate cancer and those with BPH. (Chapter 6 discusses CoQ_{10} in greater detail.) Royal jelly is a salivary secretion of honeybees that is rich in amino acids, B vitamins, and other nutrients. It has been used to support functioning of the sex organs and to treat sterility. Adding the cruciferous vegetables, such as broccoli and cauliflower and other green and orange vegetables, to the diet can also help.

See Appendix B for specific supplement guidelines for treating and preventing cancer and other prostate problems.

Get Your Yearly Checkup

Remember to have a rectal exam yearly after the age of forty, as well as an annual PSA after age fifty, or age forty if you're at high risk. And don't forget that the PSA may not be definitive. Additionally, see your doctor if any of the following symptoms develop:

• Lumps in the prostate and testicles

• Painful, weak, or interrupted urination

• Thickening or excess fluid retention in the scrotum

• Unexplained persistent low back and leg pain

PUTTING IT ALL TOGETHER

While genetics plays a role in the development of prostate cancer, diet and lifestyle appear to have more bearing. Fortunately, unlike genetics, these are factors that you can control. Research has shown that there's a correlation between external influences—including trans fat consumption, nutritional deficiencies, and environmental toxins—and prostate problems such as BPH and prostate cancer. Preventing or treating these problems is as easy as modifying the way you live, including adding nutritional and herbal supplements, such as saw palmetto extract and vital antioxidants, to your daily regimen. In addition, try to cut sugar, damaged fats, and processed foods from your diet. Choose fresh, organically grown vegetables and whole foods that are rich in fiber and antioxidants, including vitamins A, C, and E, and the minerals selenium and zinc.

6.

Keeping Your Heart Healthy

In the past three decades we have been bombarded with nutritional information and dietary mandates that should have American hearts beating to a healthy rhythm. As a nation, we are eating less meat and dietary cholesterol, smoking less cigarettes, and exercising more. So it's surprising that the incidence of heart disease has actually *increased* over the last fifteen years. And while the overall death rate from heart disease actually declined by 40 percent during that time, it still remains the leading cause of death in the United States, and the leading cause of early death in men. Statistics now tell us that, by age sixty, one in every five men will have suffered a heart attack.

More than 350,000 men will die of heart attacks this year.

All of the research and studies done on cardiovascular disease seems to have resulted in more confusion than anything else. Sorting through the daily barrage of "heart smart" information from newspapers, magazines, radio, and television can be overwhelming. By now, we all know that smoking, excess weight, lack of exercise, and poor eating habits are risk factors for heart disease. And many of us still believe that consumption of dietary cholesterol and saturated fats are the leading cause of clogged arteries.

We have been told that switching from butter to margarine, from real eggs to substitutes, is the wise thing to do.

Now, suddenly, we are being told that we were misinformed. Margarine is bad for the cardiovascular system, and real eggs don't raise our cholesterol levels. And cholesterol may not be the villain, as it has been portrayed. All of this contradictory advice reminds me of a poem by James Kavanaugh in which he says that after listening to all the conflicting advice from numerous nutritionists and doctors, he decided it was just easier to live on Fritos and Jack Daniels.

But don't give up hope! This chapter will assist you in sorting through the most up-to-date information on risk factors for heart disease. You will learn, once and for all, why not *all* cholesterol is bad. The information presented here will also help you understand the roles of cholesterol, sugar, insulin, drugs, environmental toxins, homocysteine, and iron overload in the development and progression of heart disease.

CHOLESTEROL: FRIEND OR FOE?

Heart disease results when blood flow through coronary arteries, which supply the heart with oxygen and nutrients, becomes restricted or blocked. This causes damage to the heart muscle, resulting in a heart attack. Often—but not always—heart attacks result from hardening of the arteries, known as *atherosclerosis,* a condition in which plaque, containing cholesterol and other materials, builds up in the arteries. Atherosclerosis is a degenerative condition affecting many people in our country, including young people. A 1993 study based on autopsies of 1,532 teenagers and young adults found that all of them had fatty patches in their aortas and 59 percent had heart disease.

It has become popular for us to blame cholesterol for all heart problems and to avoid cholesterol-containing foods in an effort to prevent or treat the problem. There are, in fact, many holes in this theory. Cholesterol has been associated with heart disease without question. Mosquitoes have been associated with stagnant water. But mosquitoes do not cause water to be stagnant any more than cholesterol causes plaque to build up in the arteries. Many feel that cholesterol deposits actually result from the body's efforts to repair already existing arterial damage.

Cholesterol enters our body through dietary sources, from animal products such as meat and eggs. However, the body also produces its own cholesterol. In fact, 80 percent of this substance is manufactured in the liver and brain. And it's contained in nearly every cell. *Our bodies produce cholesterol because it is essential to maintain our health.* The major functions of cholesterol include:

- Construction and repair of cell walls.

- Insulation of nerve fibers.

- Production of adrenal hormones such as cortisone, which is released in response to stress.

- Production of bile acids, which break up fats for absorption.

- Synthesis of male and female hormones.

- Vitamin D synthesis (sunlight turns cholesterol into vitamin D).

Cholesterol also has antioxidant properties and, as such, it helps to fight disease-causing free radicals.

Deficiency of cholesterol has been associated with a number of conditions, including anemia, acute infection, excess thyroid function, autoimmune disorders, and cancer. The fact is, drugs that artificially lower cholesterol can cause a number of cancers. So when it comes to cholesterol, too little can be just as harmful as too much. Again, balance is the key.

Dr. Cass Ingram (*PPNF Nutritional Journal,* Vol 15, #1–2, 1991) compiled a list of the causes of high and low cholesterol. They are as follows:

Causes of High Cholesterol

Alcoholism
Amino-acid deficiency
Antioxidant deficiency

EFA deficiency

Excess sugar, starch, or hydrogenated/processed fats in the diet

Food allergies

Liver dysfunction

Tissue damage (due to infection, radiation, free radicals)

Causes of Low Cholesterol

Adrenal stress

Cholesterol-lowering drugs

Chronic hepatitis

Immune-system decline

Liver infection/disease

Manganese deficiency

Street drugs

Cholesterol is actually a lubricant that is meant to keep the blood "oily" so it can flow freely through the blood vessels. However, when inorganic mineral deposits collect on artery walls, cholesterol may adhere to them, gradually building up into layers of artery-clogging plaques. Minerals tend to go out of solution and form deposits (in arteries and elsewhere) when the body's pH is out of balance. As you recall, pH is regulated by electrolytes. Certain trace minerals, because of their electrolyte activity, not only assure that minerals are kept in solution, but also improve digestion and metabolism of fats and encourage proper liver function.

The Role of the Liver

Liver function is critically important in cholesterol metabolism. The liver not only produces cholesterol, but also converts it into bile, and regulates its level in the blood. A healthy liver will adjust cholesterol production according to dietary intake, decreasing or increasing it as needed.

Eighty percent of the body's cholesterol is used in bile production. That bile, along with excess cholesterol, is stored in the gall bladder. When fat is present in the intestines, the gall bladder contracts, sending bile to the intestines to break down the fat. The bile is absorbed by the body in direct proportion to the amount of time it takes to pass out of the digestive tract.

Slow transit times, resulting from constipation, cause an excessive amount of bile to be reabsorbed. When bile is reabsorbed and recycled, less new bile is formed in the liver and cholesterol cannot be turned into bile at the same rate. Therefore, excessive cholesterol builds up. This theory was put forth by Dr. William Welles in his book *The Shocking Truth About Cholesterol* (1990). He states: "The real issue is bile flow, not diet."[1] One of the reasons that high-fiber foods, like oat bran, are effective in lowering cholesterol is that they decrease the reabsorption of bile salts and relieve constipation. From this perspective, factors like liver congestion and constipation and may cause cholesterol to build up.

I have found—almost without fail—that men with good elimination and healthy liver function can properly handle dietary cholesterol, as long as they are getting the nutrients necessary to metabolize it. I recommend a basic foundation for every heart-smart nutrition plan that includes the essential fatty acids, the minerals chromium and magnesium, and the B vitamins niacin and choline. These elements are largely lacking in the Standard American Diet, and the incidence of liver dysfunction and constipation is also high in our culture.

Many people are not well able to handle the cholesterol in animal foods. This does not mean, however, that they should avoid cholesterol-containing foods. What it does mean is that they should perhaps limit their intake of these foods until balance is restored in the body. In an imbalanced state, protein and fat from animal products is properly metabolized. The thing to eliminate is not the fat, nor the protein, but rather the conditions of imbalance. This calls for elimination of processed, fragmented foods and restoration of essential nutrients, especially electrolytes.

The Framingham study, in progress for more than thirty years, was designed to investigate the risk factors in heart disease. The researchers have found that the level of cholesterol in the blood does correlate with heart disease. But there is no correlation found between cholesterol in the diet and heart disease. No significant differences were found in the blood cholesterol of people who ate several eggs per week (up to twenty-four) and those who ate only a few (up to two and a half.)

UNDERSTANDING CHOLESTEROL LEVELS

Blood cholesterol does not travel through the body on its own, but must attach itself to a solid substance. In order to get cholesterol where it is needed, the liver has developed a complex system that bundles cholesterol and triglycerides—the major class of lipids in the diet and body—together into *lipoproteins.*

High-density lipoprotein (HDL) cholesterol is composed principally of lecithin, a type of phospholipid that supplies the body with choline, which is essential for liver and brain functioning. HDL carries very little fat and has more protein. Its job is to pull cholesterol back from body tissues to the liver where it's converted to bile and excreted. Low-density lipoprotein (LDL) cholesterol, on the other hand, is made up of about 50-percent cholesterol. It carries cholesterol from the liver to the parts of the body where it is needed. LDL cholesterol tends to deposit fats in the body and, if it is not controlled, these deposits can result in the development of atherosclerosis.

The latest guidelines that we've been given about cholesterol levels is that total cholesterol should be less than 200 and "good" HDL cholesterol should be greater than 35. The higher the HDL in relationship to total cholesterol, the lower the risk of heart disease. The ratio between total cholesterol and HDL cholesterol is now considered more important than just the total cholesterol alone. Optimally, the ratio of total cholesterol to HDL cholesterol should be three to one.

I remember how anxious one of my clients was when he got his most recent blood test results. Peter was a forty-five-year-old mechanic with a history of heart disease in his family. His total cholesterol was a little over 200. When I asked him what the HDL was, he said 60. I quickly put his mind at ease and congratulated him on his heart-healthy ratio.

FACTORS AFFECTING CHOLESTEROL LEVELS

Blood cholesterol levels increase or decrease according to a range of variables. Certain "bad" fats such as trans fatty acids, for instance, may raise LDL cholesterol, and at the same time lower HDL cholesterol. Insulin, too, has an impact on cholesterol levels, because the insulin response may give rise to the production of the harmful eicosanoids that we first discussed in Chapter 2. Likewise, chromium deficiency, which can cause elevated blood-sugar levels, can also cause cholesterol levels to rise.

Good Fats Versus Bad Fats

A lack of the nutrients needed for cholesterol metabolism, paired with a deficiency of antioxidant nutrients, are primary factors in the development of heart disease. The antioxidant nutrients—vitamins A, C, and E, selenium, and zinc—prevent oxidation of cholesterol. Foods left out at room temperature, or those that are fried, smoked, cured, or aged become oxidized. Oxidation gives rise to free radicals, those renegade molecules that damage blood vessel walls. The body then tries to repair the damage with cholesterol.

All processed foods—powdered milk, powdered eggs, dried custard mixes, cake mixes, aged cheeses, and smoked, dried, and aged meats, including bacon, ham, sausage, and packaged sandwich meats—give rise to free radicals. These foods can contribute significantly to the clogging of arteries.[2] It is important to understand that, while powdered eggs are to be avoided, fresh ones can be included in the diet as long as you don't fry them. Soft- or hard-boiling and poaching are the best methods for preparing eggs.

As you learned in Chapter 2, one of the most critical problems with the typical American diet is the lack of sufficient essential fatty acids. Both the omega-3 and omega-6 EFAs are involved in the regulation of cholesterol and triglycerides in the body and in the formation of many hormones. You'll recall that the higher the ratio of omega-3s to omega-6s, the less likely that a clot will obstruct an artery. Because of food processing and food choices, omega-3s are in short supply in our diet. More are needed—especially the EPA form. Increasing your intake of cold-water fish, fish oils, and flaxseed and canola oils can help you boost your omega-3 fatty-acid levels to regulate cholesterol.

Refined and man-made hydrogenated oils need to be totally eliminated from the diet, for the trans fats they form interfere with the functioning of EFAs and increase serum cholesterol. TFAs actually raise "bad" LDL cholesterol, and lower "good" HDL cholesterol. When Northern Europe's supply of hydrogenated foods was cut off during the last world war, the result was the most dramatic decline in heart disease of the century!

Insulin Strikes Again

Remember our discussion from Chapter 2 about the hormonal effects of food? The insulin response from a diet too high in carbohydrates produces harmful eicosanoids that can lead to high blood pressure, heart attack, atherosclerosis, increased fat storage, and unstable sugar levels. You learned how balancing macronutrients with the 40/30/30 plan creates a favorable hormonal response, as a result of the glucagon release triggered by the protein. Not only will this mobilize stored body fat, but the "good" eicosanoids produced will regulate the cardiovascular system.

The Balance Bar Company, makers of the Balance nutrition bar, sponsored two independent clinical studies, one at Pepperdine University and the other at Sansum Medical Research Foundation in Santa Barbara. These studies demonstrated that the 40/30/30 formula not only improves athletic performance, aids in weight loss, and is safe for people with diabetes, but also raises the levels of good HDL cholesterol. The Pepperdine University double-blind crossover study showed an increase in HDL of 13.5 points in just four weeks.[3]

I have lectured and written about the dangers of high-carbohydrate intake in several of my books. This issue has also been recognized by some progressive members of the medical profession. As quoted in *The Santa Barbara News* in December 1994, Diana L. Schwarzbein, a Santa Barbara endocrinologist, believes that:

Eating foods high in cholesterol does not increase blood cholesterol. . . . Overeating carbohydrates can lead to abnormal cholesterol levels. And foods that raise insulin levels are the ones that cause obesity, high blood pressure, high cholesterol and heart disease.

A diet high in carbohydrates is one that will put a man at risk for developing cardiovascular disease. This is especially true if that diet is made up of refined carbohydrates.

Chromium Deficiency

In the refining process, white sugar loses 93 percent of its chromium. White flour has only 23 micrograms per 100 grams of this important trace mineral, compared with the 175 micrograms per 100 grams found in whole wheat flour (if the wheat was grown in mineral-rich soil). It is well known that chromium plays an important role in sugar metabolism. What is not so well known is that it also plays a crucial part in fat metabolism.

It appears that there is a link between disorders of fat metabolism and those of sugar metabolism: practically everybody with clinical atherosclerosis of moderate severity has a mild form of diabetes. People with moderate to severe diabetes have especially severe atherosclerosis, from which most die. This association was established a number of years ago. In 1959, researchers discovered that rats with reduced glucose tolerance, or diabetes, were chromium deficient. This disorder can be prevented or cured by adding chromium to the diet. It was later established conclusively that chromium is necessary for the utilization of insulin in glucose metabolism. Subsequent animal studies indicated not only elevated blood sugar levels when chromium was deficient, but also elevated blood cholesterol levels. Both can be lowered by the addition of chromium to the diet.

When it comes to humans, chromium tends to be present in the bodies of all young people. However, according to Dr. Schroeder, author of *The Trace Elements and Man* (The Devin-üdair Company, 1973), it is not detected at all in the tissues of 15 to 23 percent of

Americans over fifty. Chromium is present, however, in 98.5 percent of foreigners over fifty. Furthermore, no chromium was found in the aortas of people who died from coronary artery disease, while it was present in those who died of other causes. These findings highlight the importance of including chromium in the diet for the prevention of heart disease. Good sources of chromium include brewer's yeast, brown rice, cheese, clams, corn oil, grapes, honey, meat, raisins, and whole-grain cereals. (Refer to Chapter 3 for a more detailed discussion of chromium.)

In view of these findings, we would be wise to limit our intake of refined foods, or better yet, to eliminate them entirely—especially white sugar and white flour. Many individuals following the gospel of the low-fat, high-carbohydrate diet over the last decade have overdosed on sugar.

What the Evidence Shows

People around the world enjoy good health, free of heart disease, until they either migrate to Westernized cities or adopt a Western diet, heavy in sugar-laden, processed foods. Several Mediterranean societies have also been free of cardiovascular disease, despite a diet that is up to 70-percent fat. Among people whose native diet consists of a high percentage of animal fat are the Yemini Jews, the Eskimos, and the Masai tribesmen of Africa.

Over thirty years ago, Ancel Keys, Ph.D., discovered that people living in the southern European countries had a very low rate of heart disease. It was especially low among the people of the Greek island, Crete—90 percent lower than the United States—despite the fact that 40 percent of their diet was composed of fat. Olive oil, a monounsaturated fat, was their primary source of fat, with only 8 percent of the calories coming from saturated fats.

Another group of people with a very low incidence of heart disease are the Japanese from Kohama Island. These people have something in common with the people of Crete—they both have a high dietary intake of linolenic acid, an omega-3 EFA. The Cretans get their linolenic acid from walnuts and purslane, a thick-leaved "weedy" plant used in salads, while the Japanese get theirs from soybean products and rapeseed (canola) oil.

French researchers took a group of 605 patients who had one heart attack, and placed half of them on a typical Cretan diet. They ate bread, grains, vegetables, fruit, poultry, fish, and some cheese, and used only olive and canola oil for cooking. No butter or margarine was used, but rather a spread rich in omega-3 essential fatty acids. The other half of the patients were placed on the American Heart Association diet, high in polyunsaturated fats and low in cholesterol and saturated fats. Total fat was restricted to 30 percent, with saturated fat limited to 10 percent. Their progress was charted over a twenty-seven-month period, during which time the cholesterol levels, blood pressures, and weight of people in both groups remained about the same.

Interestingly, there was a marked difference in the number of patients having a second heart attack and surviving it. Of the individuals on the American Heart Association diet, thirty-three had heart attacks, and sixteen people died as a result of heart attacks. On the other hand, of the people following the Mediterranean diet, only eight suffered heart attacks, and three individuals died from heart attacks.[4]

The advantages of the Mediterranean diet were so obvious that the study was prematurely ended. The patients on the AHA diet were put on the Cretan diet. By the completion of the study, those on the Cretan diet showed concentrations of linolenic acid in the blood that were near to that of the natives of Crete and Kohma. This study is significant in that it demonstrates that establishing omega-3 EFA sufficiency is more important than lowering cholesterol. It is not necessary that we adopt a Mediterranean diet, though it may be most beneficial to those of Southern European ancestry, but we do want to get plenty of omega-3 fatty acids in our diet.

TAME YOUR SWEET TOOTH

Sugar is eight times as concentrated as flour and much more harmful. The refining process has robbed it of trace minerals and many other nutrients, including the family of B vitamins. In the absence of B vitamins, carbohydrate metabolism can't take place. When carbohydrates aren't properly broken down, they ferment in the system, adding a toxic burden to the body. Sugar is, of course, a carbohydrate. When we consume sugar in its refined form, in which none of the nutrients needed to metabolize it are present, the body must rob its storehouses to obtain these nutrients. As the storehouses become depleted, degenerative diseases develop.

The average American consumes over 138 pounds of sugar and high fructose corn syrup per year. That breaks down to over four dozen teaspoons daily per person! Only one-fourth of that amount is consumed at the table and for cooking. The rest is found in our foods. And it's not just in the obvious foods like cookies, cake, candy, and ice cream. Sugar is also hidden in ketchup, salad dressings, canned soups, peanut butter, luncheon meats, and canned and frozen vegetables. Even cigarettes, cigars, and pipe tobacco contain sugar! Used in curing tobacco, sugar contributes to the addictive qualities of tobacco products. *Read labels.* There are many forms of sugar and many names for it. Avoid foods containing corn syrup and any containing ingredients that end in "ose."

As sugar consumption increases, so does the incidence of heart disease. A professor of nutrition and dietetics at Queen Elizabeth College of London University found the following associations between deaths from heart disease or heart attack (per 10,000 people) and the amount of sugar they consumed per year: 20 pounds per person resulted in 60 deaths; 120 pounds per person resulted in 300 deaths; and 150 pounds per person resulted in 750 deaths.[5]

Sugar raises triglyceride, cholesterol, and insulin levels, and raises blood pressure as well. Tests at Brookhaven National Laboratory found that patients on a high-sugar, low-fat diet had triglyceride levels two to five times greater than those on a low-sugar, high-fat diet. High sugar intake also contributes to obesity. These are all risk factors for the development of heart disease. But that's not all. Sugar has also been linked with birth defects, cancer, diabetes, gallstones, hypoglycemia, kidney damage, learning disabilities, migraine headaches, premature aging, reduced immunity, and tooth decay.

Our liking for that sweet taste may have been nature's way of prompting us to include fruits and vegetables in our diet. Back when they were rich in minerals, these foods had a sweet taste. Because of their fiber content, naturally sweet foods delay the release of sugar into the bloodstream and their minerals assist in its utilization. On the other hand, consuming sugar by itself, or any of the concentrated sugars—such as honey, barley malt, rice syrup, maple syrup, and molasses—triggers an immediate insulin response and all of the attendant negative consequences.

All of these sweeteners are refined products. Even "raw" sugar is only white sugar to which molasses has been added. While these foods are somewhat more nutritious than white sugar, they all raise cholesterol and triglycerides, depress immune activity, and contribute to yeast overgrowth, which can cause fatigue and a variety of mental symptoms. Excess sugar can also block the manufacture of good prostaglandins from essential fatty acids.

Fructose: The Natural Alternative?

Many people consider fructose to be a healthy alternative to refined sugar because it's a "natural" sweetener found in fruit. Over the past fifteen years, consumption of high fructose corn syrup has tripled, going from 19 pounds per person in 1980 to 56 pounds in 1994. During that same period, sugar consumption actually decreased. High fructose corn syrup is widely used by food manufacturers in soft drinks, baked goods, jellies, jams, syrups, and ketchup. Even health food stores deal in fructose, sold in its crystalline form and as an ingredient in concentrated fruit juices.

Since fructose has a low glycemic index rating—meaning that it does not convert quickly to blood sugar, or raise insulin levels rapidly—it has been recommended by some for people with diabetes. However, this recommendation is invalid. The liver is the only organ that can metabolize fructose. A high-fructose diet puts a strain on the liver similar to that of alcohol consumption. While every cell in the body can metabolize glucose, the liver must convert fructose into glucose before it enters insulin pathways. For these reasons, fructose should be avoided by diabetics.

Another strike against fructose is that it elevates "bad" LDL cholesterol, thereby increasing the risk of heart disease. The U.S. Department of Agriculture study found in 1993 that consuming as little as two to three soft drinks with high fructose corn syrup daily can elevate LDL levels.

A warning about switching to diet sodas: Diet sodas contain *aspartame*, sold under the trade names of NutraSweet or Equal. Although there is no evidence linking it to cholesterol levels, aspartame has its own set of health problems. Severe anxiety attacks, confusion, convulsions, decreased vision, depression, dizziness, extreme irritability, headaches, nausea, numbing of hand and feet, palpitations, marked personality changes, and ringing in the ears have all been associated with ingestion of aspartame. Eighty to eighty-five percent of consumer complaints to the FDA have involved aspartame. And aspartame is not only found in diet soda. Over 1,200 products, including children's vitamins, drugs, baked goods, laxatives, and chewing gum now contain aspartame.*

THE HOMOCYSTEINE FACTOR

In a revolutionary new book entitled *The Homocysteine Revolution* (Keats, 1997), Harvard-trained physician and researcher Kilmer S. McCully suggests that elevated levels of a potentially toxic amino acid called homocysteine is a more potent risk factor than cholesterol in predicting heart disease. His theory points to our vitamin-B depleted food supply as the underlying cause behind the heart disease epidemic. Three vitally important B vitamins—B_6, B_{12}, and folic acid—are lost from our food supply due to processing and packaging. Consequently, a deficiency of these vitamins and the amino acid methionine elevates levels of homocysteine resulting

---

* The Aspartame Consumer Safety Network has volumes of available information on the dangers of aspartame. Write to: P.O. Box 780634, Dallas, TX 75378, or call: 214–352–4268.

from the normal metabolic breakdown of proteins in the system. In combination with the "bad" LDL cholesterol, homocysteine damages the arterial walls and plaque can build up in the heart. Stroke and blood clots in the legs or lungs have also been tied to elevated homocysteine levels.

The good news is that vitamin B_{12} and folic acid can convert homocysteine to the harmless essential amino acid methionine. In addition, vitamin B_6 helps to decrease homocysteine levels by converting homocysteine into cysteine for excretion from the body.

I suggest that all of my clients have their homocysteine levels tested on a yearly basis. There are now homocysteine formulas on the market that contain higher amounts of vitamins B_6, B_{12}, and folic acid. According to Dr. Ronald L. Hoffman, in his book *Intelligent Medicine* (Fireside, 1997), the following daily supplements are recommended for people with elevated homocysteine levels:

Folic acid: 5 milligrams daily

Vitamin B_6: 100 milligrams daily

Vitamin B_{12}: 1,000 micrograms (1 milligram) daily

With proper vitamin supplementation, many people find it easy to reduce their elevated homocysteine levels.

IRON OVERLOAD

Another heart disease culprit, iron overload, may be as new to you as it was to me. Just as I was finishing this book, I got a call from my uncle, Jack Kriwitsky, who insisted I meet with him and a friend for dinner that night. At dinner, I met Jack Fox, my uncle's friend who had just returned from a conference in Florida on iron overload. He gave me a book entitled *The Iron Elephant* (Vida, 1992). Much of what I learned about iron is from this book. I also learned that Jack Fox had become so interested in the iron problem because of his lady friend who had the problem and discovered it quite by accident.

Plain and simple, iron can be a hidden killer that adversely affects the heart under certain circumstances. High levels of iron in the body have been linked with heart disease and hypertension, as well as with headaches, liver disorders, arthritis, diabetes, and cancer. A five-year study conducted in Finland followed 1,900 men who had no clinical evidence of heart disease when the study began in 1984.[6] The researchers measured the amount of ferritin, a protein that binds iron in the blood. They found that for each 1-percent increase in the amount of ferritin in the blood, there was a more than 4-percent increase in heart attack risk. A ferritin level of 200 micrograms or greater more than doubled the relative risk of heart attack. Typical ferritin levels for adult males are from 100 to 150 micrograms. Next to smoking, the study found ferritin levels to be the strongest risk factor for heart attack. LDL levels alone were not found to be a significant risk factor, but they were significant when paired with elevated iron. Another study found iron in atherosclerotic plaques in humans. And iron promotes oxidation of LDL cholesterol.

These findings underscore the importance for men of excluding iron supplements from their diet unless a need for the mineral is demonstrated through laboratory analysis. And men must also make sure that the iron they put into their bodies is from organic sources, or bioavailable, so that it stays in solution and does not contribute to plaque formation. To assure this, body pH must be normalized through electrolyte balance and a balanced diet. Since meat is high in bioavailable iron, excessive consumption of it can cause a build-up of the mineral in the body, especially if pH is off balance.

Surprisingly, new research indicates that many people suffer from iron overload caused by a genetic condition known as *hereditary hemochromatosis* (HH). People with normal iron metabolism absorb no more than the amount of iron needed daily, while those with HH absorb it excessively, to toxic levels. Once absorbed, iron is not excreted. The only way iron levels can be lowered is through blood loss. Once thought to be extremely rare, HH is proving to be quite prevalent, especially among Caucasians, affecting 2 of every 400 people.

Over a million Americans carry the gene for hemochromatosis. Roberta Crawford was one of them. It took her twenty-six years and four doctors to get a correct diagnosis. During this period of time, she was misdiagnosed, as many are, with anemia and given more iron. Her symptoms included headaches, joint pain, diarrhea, heart irregularities, and heavy menstrual bleeding. After her ordeal, Crawford formed the Iron Overload Diseases Association and wrote *The Iron Elephant* to help educate the public about the problems associated with iron overload.*

Symptoms of excess iron can also include abdominal pain, anemia, fatigue, lack of mental clarity, low immunity, and a gray or bronze tint to the skin. Over time, the accumulation of iron in the system can cause organ damage, resulting in such conditions as arthritis, cancer, cirrhosis, diabetes, heart disease, impotence, premature menopause, and sterility.

Many people, like Crawford, are misdiagnosed, as doctors commonly make the faulty assumption that anemia is caused only by low iron levels—without doing the proper testing. Anemia can be diagnosed with a fingerprick test and hemoglobin count, but without further laboratory analysis, the cause of the anemia cannot be ascertained with certainty. While low iron levels can cause anemia, iron overload can cause it too. The most effective tests to screen for HH are those that measure serum iron (SI) concentration, the total iron-binding capacity (TIBC), and the stored iron or ferritin.

Once HH is diagnosed, it is important that family members be tested, since it can be passed on genetically. Prognosis for HH is good, especially if it's detected early before organ damage results. For this reason, blood profiles are recommended for those men showing symptoms that may indicate HH.

Iron overload should be considered a major risk factor in heart disease, second only to cigarette smoking. Excess iron causes the oxidation of LDL, promoting the formation of plaque in the arteries. Becoming a frequent blood donor is the main therapy for iron overload.

---

* You can contact the Iron Overload Diseases Association at 433 Westwind Drive, Dept. W, North Palm Beach, FL 33408 (407–840–8512).

ENVIRONMENTAL TOXINS AND THE HEART

Our environment—the air we breathe, the food we eat, the water we drink—is becoming increasingly contaminated. Among the pollutants are a class of toxic minerals known as heavy metals, including lead, cadmium, aluminum, and mercury. None of these metals belong in our bodies (except for a minute amount of aluminum), but have found their way there through our polluted food, air, and water supplies.

Heavy metals have been linked with heart disease, among other disorders. Lead toxicity is associated with cardiovascular dysfunction, arteriosclerosis, and atherosclerosis; aluminum toxicity can paralyze the heart; mercury—even in small amounts—can damage the heart, as well as other organs; and cadmium toxicity gives rise to hypertension. This happens because cadmium replaces zinc in the arterial walls, leading to reduced flexibility and strength in the arteries. A buildup in arterial plaque results, as the body coats the arteries in an effort to prevent formation of aneurysms.

HEART DISEASE

Cardiomyopathy is a generalized term, pertaining to myocardia, or heart muscle, disease. The term encompasses congestive heart failure (CHF), atherosclerosis, and high blood pressure, also known as hypertension. There's evidence that cardiomyopathy results from selenium deficiency. This was demonstrated in 1972, when Keshan disease, which has plagued the Keshan Province of the People's Republic of China since 1930, was found to be identical to mulberry heart disease in pigs, known to be caused by a selenium deficiency. As it turns out, the soil in Keshan Province is almost totally lacking in selenium.

One of the many functions of selenium in the human body is the protection of the cellular membranes of both skeletal and cardiac muscle fibers from free-radical damage. A selenium deficiency is intensified by exercise and by a high intake of polyunsaturated fats. This important trace mineral is added to commercial food for pets, and laboratory and farm animals, but not to food meant for human consumption. So the pigs may not be getting mulberry heart disease anymore, but we are!

The next few pages will explore two distinct problems—congestive heart failure and hypertension—in more detail.

Congestive Heart Failure

While the death rate for heart disease has been decreasing, the number of cases of congestive heart failure (CHF) have increased. According to American Heart Association statistics, the number of people hospitalized for the disease more than doubled between 1979 and 1992, jumping from 377,000 to 822,000. It is the most common cause of hospitalization for people over sixty-five, with 50,000 people dying from it each year, and cost of care exceeding $50 billion annually.

The American Heart Association describes CHF as a condition in which the heart becomes weakened, unable to pump out all the blood that flows through it. According to Dr. Bruce West, CHF would more appropriately be called "beriberi of the heart."[7] Beriberi is a disease caused by deficiency of B vitamins, especially B_1, or thiamine. Symptoms of this deficiency disease include nerve conductivity problems, weakness, and muscle paralysis. Dr. West draws the parallel to CHF, describing it as a "problem of poor nerve conductivity to the heart, an almost paralyzing weakness of the heart muscle and the resultant failure of the heart muscle to be able to pump out blood."[8]

According to Dr. West, vitamin B_4, which has not been synthesized, nor recognized by the FDA, together with B_1, are vitally important for proper heart muscle function. He emphasizes the fact that all of the B vitamins are linked together by thousands of plant chemicals known as phytochemicals, most of which have not been synthesized or even identified. Phytochemicals are needed to activate vitamins and minerals, and they are absent in isolated vitamins produced in the laboratory. We must look to whole foods as a source of supply. The alternative is to use a B-complex supplement made from food and plant sources, one that is processed in such a way as to maintain the phytochemicals. The B vitamins are found in brewer's yeast, liver, and whole-grain cereals. Vitamin B_1 is also found in egg yolks, fish, fowl, legumes, meat, and nuts.

Julian Whitaker, M.D., has observed that thirty years ago patients with CHF invariably had a history of heart attack that had inflicted damage upon the heart muscle. Today, some CHF patients have no history of heart attack. Dr. Whitaker believes that the factor responsible for this and for the escalation of CHF over the last few decades is the "overuse of medications called beta blockers."[9] Beta blockers are used to lower blood pressure. They do so by blocking the heart's ability to respond to epinephrine and adrenaline, two hormones that stimulate and elevate both blood pressure and pulse rate. Basically, these drugs lower blood pressure by weakening the heart.

Dr. Whitaker believes that, while beta blockers are useful for temporary relief of symptoms, long-term use can lead to congestive heart failure. His belief is supported by multiple references in the *Physicians Desk Reference*, which doctors use to prescribe drugs. The PDR points to possible cardiac side effects including heart failure from long-term use of beta-blockers such as Lopressor.

Calcium channel blockers, another class of drugs commonly prescribed for high blood pressure, are also associated with an increase in death from heart disease—a 60-percent increase. The mineral magnesium works better than these drugs as a calcium-blocking agent to prevent spasm of the coronary arteries—and it has no side effects.

Separate studies have found that supplementation with taurine, a nonessential amino acid,[10] and the mineral potassium[11] can be useful in the treatment of CHF. A deficiency of muscle potassium could not, however, be corrected if magnesium deficiency was also present.

Hypertension

Hypertension is an abnormal elevation of blood pressure that can lead to heart and kidney diseases or stroke. It affects one out of four men. Actual physical ailments such as kidney infection, obstruction of a kidney artery, adrenal disorder, or constriction of the aorta account for about 10 percent of the cases. These conditions can usually be corrected. For the majority of people, however, the exact cause of hypertension is not known. The condition is then referred to as *essential hypertension.* A major factor associated with hypertension is atherosclerosis, which obstructs the flow of blood through arteries. Stress is also an important factor, for it causes contraction of arterial walls.

When blood pressure is high, the body is out of balance. Drugs used to lower pressure won't correct the basic imbalance, which is an electrolyte imbalance, and indeed can further disturb it. A possible side effect of hypertension drugs is cardiac problems. Diuretics are the most commonly prescribed medication for hypertension, and they are the safest. But you should be aware that diuretics can rob the body of minerals essential to heart function. As Dr. Earl Mindell explains in his *Joy of Health* newsletter (April 1995, page 3):

> *Most diuretics lower blood pressure by preventing the kidneys from returning sodium to the blood, which increases the volume of urine. The result is to reduce the volume of fluid in the blood and in other cells of the body. Unfortunately, as the urine carries sodium out of the body, it takes other minerals salts with it, most importantly potassium and magnesium—two minerals that are essential to your heart health.*

Since one of the purposes of taking diuretics is to reduce sodium levels, a sodium-restricted diet is recommended for people with hypertension. Sodium intake can be reduced just by avoiding packaged and processed foods. There's no need to avoid foods that are naturally high in sodium, such as celery—in fact, it has been found that there's a substance in celery that can relax the walls of blood vessels. Regular table salt, which is highly processed and devoid of trace minerals, should be eliminated entirely. It can be replaced with a totally unrefined, mineral-rich salt such as Celtic Sea salt* used in moderation. This type of salt will not cause fluid retention. Most sea salts found in health food stores are processed to some degree and should be avoided.

* Celtic Sea salt is available through the Grain and Salt Society (916–872–5800).

Salt restriction will not lower blood pressure if potassium levels are low, which is most often the case with people who take diuretics. Symptoms of potassium deficiency include constipation, insomnia, irregular heartbeat, muscle cramps, nervous disorders, and weakness. The level of this important mineral can be increased by eating potassium-rich foods such as fruits, vegetables, lean meats, legumes, sunflower seeds, and whole grains. Drinking fresh fruit and vegetable juices is an excellent way to get plenty of potassium. If you take diuretics to control hypertension, you should take in around 2,000 milligrams of potassium daily from food sources.

Diuretics not only cause potassium loss but also the excretion of other minerals such as calcium and magnesium. Inadequate levels of calcium, magnesium, and potassium can cause contraction of blood vessels, resulting in elevated blood pressure—which puts us right back where we started! To replace these minerals, I recommend regular use of a good multimineral formula in conjunction with the Trace-Lyte electrolyte formula. Long-term use of diuretics can result in impaired glucose tolerance if potassium and chromium aren't replaced.

Spending more time outside in the sun can help to increase vitamin D levels. This, together with increased intake of potassium and calcium, will cause the body to excrete more sodium. Vitamin C and bioflavonoids can help maintain or restore the health of blood vessels strained by the increased pressure they're under.

Weight loss can favorably influence blood pressure. In fact, for every 2 pounds of weight lost, blood pressure should drop 1 point in both systolic (top number) and diastolic (bottom number) readings. Most people with hypertension are overweight, weighing an average of 29 pounds more than people with normal blood pressure. Even 5 pounds of excess body weight can contribute to high blood pressure. Weight loss can be achieved without dieting, simply by following the 40/30/30 eating plan.

Regular exercise is also helpful in reducing blood pressure. Individuals who exercise are 34 percent less likely to develop hypertension than those who don't. Strenuous exercise is not necessary. Dr. Mindell tells us that "just a brisk half-hour walk three to four times a week can lower blood pressure by 3 to 15 points in just three months."[12]

Hypertension, like diabetes, is associated with insulin. Both conditions can be caused by insulin resistance. In insulin resistance, the pancreas (even in the person with diabetes) produces plenty of insulin—sometimes too much. The problem is that the insulin just isn't getting to the cells because its entry is blocked by fat. In addition to avoiding the "bad" fats—such as trans fats, refined oils, or too much unsaturated fat—and replacing them with EFAs, insulin resistance can be prevented or corrected by reducing carbohydrates, which trigger the insulin response.

The trace element vanadium inhibits the synthesis of cholesterol and, given in large doses in the form of vanadyl sulfate, can eliminate diabetes and certain forms of high blood pressure. It appears to do this by making cells more responsive to insulin. The intriguing thing is that improvement is sustained even after supplementation is discontinued, according to research studies.

Apart from the traditional risk factors associated with hypertension—excess weight, stress, lack of exercise, smoking, and poor diet—we can add "exposure to environmental toxins," such as cadmium, to our list.

SUPPLEMENTS FOR A HEALTHY HEART

Heart problems are not inevitable. By making changes to your diet and implementing a program of regular exercise, you can keep your heart strong and healthy and greatly reduce your chances of developing heart disease. For example, nutritional supplements such as carnitine and coenzyme Q_{10} can help regulate triglyceride and cholesterol levels. Magnesium is well known as a "heart-smart" mineral, but one that the majority of men are deficient in. Likewise, all men need to make sure they take in sufficient amounts of powerful antioxidants such as vitamin E, superoxide dismutase, and glutathione peroxidase.

Carnitine

Carnitine is a vitamin-like substance once considered to be a nonessential amino acid. The body can synthesize carnitine from the essential amino acids lysine and methionine. The conversion cannot take place, however, without adequate iron and vitamin C. Higher levels of carnitine are found in men's blood than in women's, suggesting that men have a greater need for it.

Carnitine stimulates fat metabolism, regulates triglyceride levels, increases HDL cholesterol, and decreases LDL cholesterol. It can be of potential value for a number of heart disorders. When carnitine levels are normalized through supplementation, the heart can better use its limited oxygen supply. In addition, it has recently been demonstrated that carnitine can help protect cells from damage wrought by free radicals, though it is not actually an antioxidant. Rather than neutralizing free radicals, carnitine helps cells recover from free-radical damage.

Dietary sources of carnitine include muscle and organ meats, dairy products, and legumes. It is not present in vegetable protein, however, and vegetarians may be deficient due to low levels of the precursor, lysine, in the diet.

Coenzyme Q_{10}

Like carnitine, coenzyme Q_{10}, or CoQ_{10}, is another vitamin-like compound that can be synthesized by the body. It's a substance found in all body cells, with the greatest concentration in the liver and the heart, but tissue levels decrease with age. CoQ_{10} plays a major role in energy production in the body and a deficiency of it can cause or aggravate many conditions, including heart disease, diabetes, and periodontal disease. CoQ_{10} can lower triglycerides and total cholesterol, while raising "good" HDL cholesterol. It appears to be useful as a weight-loss aid due to its ability to stimulate the mitochondria and increase the fat-burning process.

The heart may be particularly vulnerable to CoQ_{10} deficiency because it contains the most metabolically active tissues in the body. A CoQ_{10} deficiency has been demonstrated in up to 75 percent of myocardial biopsies in patients with various heart diseases. Conditions such as angina (heart pain), mitral valve prolapse, high blood pressure, and congestive heart failure can benefit from

CoQ_{10} supplementation. A University of Texas study using coenzyme Q_{10} with CHF patients found that 78 percent improved and their survival rate was higher than those receiving standard treatment.

Good food sources of CoQ_{10} are meat, some types of fish, and certain vegetable oils. Other good sources include rice bran, wheat germ, soy and other beans.

Magnesium

Every man that I work with is directed to take extra magnesium. I firmly believe that magnesium deficiency is the cause of many of our current maladies, including heart disease.

Magnesium is the second most common mineral in our cells. It plays a major role in protecting the heart. Deficiency of this important mineral has been linked to hypertension, arrhythmias, and CHF. Insufficient magnesium can cause coronary artery spasms that reduce blood and oxygen flow to the heart, resulting in a heart attack. It has been found that individuals who died suddenly from heart attacks had very low levels of magnesium in their hearts. Death from ischemic heart disease, caused by obstruction of arteries, is more common in areas where soil and water have low levels of magnesium. It has also been shown that magnesium is needed for the body to use insulin properly.

A recent Gallup survey found that 72 percent of adult male Americans fail to meet the 350-milligram Recommended Daily Allowance for magnesium. The survey also showed that magnesium consumption decreases with age. Low levels of magnesium not only increase the risk of developing high blood pressure and heart disease, but also increase susceptibility to insomnia, muscle cramps, diabetes, kidney stones, and cancer.

Compounding the problem of low magnesium intake is the high calcium intake of Americans. Magnesium should optimally be taken in equal proportion to calcium. Americans have been urged to eat more dairy products as a source of calcium, and we're doing so, much to our detriment. Dairy products contain nine times as much calcium as magnesium.

Early man adapted to an environment rich in magnesium but lacking in calcium by developing mechanisms for storing calcium. Our bodies still store calcium more efficiently than magnesium, so we don't need as much of it in our diet as we've been led to believe. What little magnesium we do consume in the Standard American Diet is depleted by a diet high in sugar and alcohol, which increases magnesium excretion through the urine.

Magnesium is abundant in whole foods—leafy greens, legumes, nuts, seeds, tofu, whole grains, and sea vegetables. However, refined foods, which are so abundant in the typical American's diet, lack adequate levels of this valuable mineral. We can get ample calcium in our diets without including dairy products that are not well absorbed due to their low magnesium content and their high phosphorus content.

Other Heart-Smart Nutrients

Since the oxidation of harmful LDL cholesterol is proving to be an important contributing factor in heart disease, antioxidant nutrients become important weapons in the fight against the disease. Flavonoids are powerful antioxidants found in fruits and vegetables. A five-year study involving 500 men in the Netherlands found that those who consumed the most flavonoid-rich foods were half as likely to have a heart attack or die from coronary disease as those eating the least amount of flavonoids.

Vitamin E

One study on vitamin E involved 39,910 healthy men. It began in 1986 and lasted for four years. During that period of time, 667 of the men developed coronary artery disease. The study found that those men with the highest vitamin E intake had 40-percent less risk of coronary disease compared with those men with the lowest intakes. Risk reduction was seen only for men taking in at least 100 international units (IU) per day, and the use of supplements for at least two years seemed to be necessary to achieve this protection.

Another study interviewed patients following angioplasty—a procedure in which blocked coronary arteries are dilated—and found that those who regularly took vitamin E experienced restenosis, the reoccurrence of blood vessel narrowing, at a rate of only 15.8 percent compared with a rate of 30.7 percent in those not taking the vitamin.

B Complex Vitamins

I've already mentioned some of the B vitamin family members that play an important role in protecting the heart—B_1, B_4, and choline, which is necessary for fat metabolism. The body's fat metabolism can be impaired by a severe deficiency of biotin, a B vitamin needed for the metabolism of carbohydrates, fats, and protein. Vitamins B_6 and B_{12} and folic acid are also helpful for keeping homocysteine levels down.

Niacin (vitamin B_3) has been used for many years to treat high cholesterol and elevated triglyceride levels. High doses of niacin can cause flushing of the skin, itching, upset stomach, and increased levels of blood glucose, uric acid, and liver enzymes. For this reason, you should take large doses of this vitamin under the supervision of a health-care professional. Do not use niacin if you have a history of gout, liver dysfunction, or diabetes.

Antioxidant Enzymes

Important antioxidant enzymes, such as superoxide dismutase (SOD) and glutathione peroxidase, scavenge free radicals seven to ten times faster than antioxidant vitamins and minerals. Supplemental antioxidant enzymes, however, have low bioavailability and can be quite costly. Good food sources of the antioxidant enzymes are alfalfa, barley, bee pollen, wheat grass juice, and wheat sprouts.

A true electrolyte formula, which includes trace minerals in a crystalloid form, will also enhance this ability. Trace minerals, including manganese and zinc, are needed for the production of SOD factors. Glutathione peroxidase is also mineral-dependent—it requires selenium. Both glutathione peroxidase and SOD are normally present in large amounts in heart tissue to protect it from oxidative damage.

Selenium

In humans, a link has been found between selenium and heart disease. People found to have overt selenium deficiencies have also been found to suffer from heart problems that respond to selenium supplementation. Selenium is the mineral activator of the vitamin E complex. The mineral works together with vitamin E to protect the heart. A deficiency of either nutrient can be damaging, but a deficiency of both is observed to produce more severe oxidative damage.

Bromelain

We've heard from the aspirin people that an aspirin a day will keep clotting away. And while there have been studies showing that aspirin can be helpful in preventing clotting that can lead to heart attacks, aspirin can have serious side effects, such as bleeding of the stomach lining, when taken regularly. Recent studies link aspirin to macular degeneration, the number-one cause of blindness in people over fifty-five.

Fortunately, there's a safe, natural alternative to aspirin for achieving antiblood-clotting results. It is an extract from pineapple called bromelain. Research shows that bromelain breaks down arteriosclerotic plaques and relieves angina pectoris through enzymatic action. In one study, fourteen patients with angina were given 400 to 1,000 milligrams daily of bromelain and all were asymptomatic within ninety days—some in as few as four days, depending on severity. Systemic enzyme therapy can also be used to improve blood fluidity and circulation.

Pycnogenol

Another extremely potent antioxidant is Pycnogenol, which comes from pine tree bark. Studies show that it is completely nontoxic and highly bioavailable. Rather than being a specific nutrient, Pycnogenol is actually a group of substances called *proanthocyanidins* found in a particular type of flavonoid or bioflavonoid. This antioxidant has been found to scavenge free radicals 50 percent more effectively than vitamin E and 20 percent more effectively than vitamin C. Proanthocyanidins greatly increase vitamin C activity, strengthening collagen in the blood vessels and increasing capillary resiliency. This, in turn, improves circulation.

Dr. David White at the University of Nottingham in England found that proanthocyanidins prevent the oxidation of LDL cholesterol. While vitamin E scavenges free radicals only in fatty areas of the body, and vitamin C scavenges them only in watery areas, Pycnogenol scavenges them in both locations. It also has anti-inflammatory activity.

Herbs

Antioxidants and flavonoids help to improve circulation, strengthen blood vessels, and decrease clotting, thereby lowering the risk of atherosclerosis, heart disease, and stroke. Certain herbs contain these compounds. Most notable of them is hawthorn, a member of the rose family that contains anthocyanidins and proanthocyanidins, which give the plant its antioxidant properties. Hawthorn decreases cholesterol, inhibits atherosclerotic plaque buildup, lowers blood pressure, and dilates coronary vessels, which improves blood flow and increases blood supply to the heart muscle. This herb has also been shown to increase the force of the heart's contraction and prevent arrythmias. Although it works well with many heart medications, you should not use hawthorn if you take beta blockers.

Another herb that has been demonstrated to decrease cholesterol and triglyceride levels is garlic. These findings have been the result of studies on animals and humans conducted for over thirty years. Consuming 600 milligrams per day (half of a clove) of garlic powder for two weeks reduced significantly the susceptibility of fats in the blood to oxidation. Garlic has powerful antioxidant properties and can lower cholesterol by at least 10 percent in less than one month. It also has the ability to prevent blood from clotting. Be aware, however, that raw garlic can lower blood sugar.

Cayenne can play an important role in supporting heart function. It has been used traditionally by herbalists as a crisis herb in coronary and other emergencies. Cayenne is also useful when taken on a regular basis (a quarter teaspoon taken three times daily) to stimulate circulation and prevent heart attacks and stroke. It also helps prevent arthritis, colds, flu, headaches, and indigestion. Both cayenne and garlic have been used successfully to lower blood pressure in hypertension.

START TAKING CHARGE

Heart disease is a product of modern "civilized" society—stressful lifestyles and diets consisting heavily of devitalized foods create the conditions for its development. As with all of the illnesses discussed so far, changes in your dietary habits are essential for improving your heart's health.

As you've read, high dietary cholesterol does not necessarily correlate with an increase in heart disease. Increased sugar consumption does. What you need to do now is switch your focus. Don't concentrate on selecting foods with those "no cholesterol" labels, but instead start keeping an eye out for hidden sugars in prepackaged foods and condiments.

The saying that "the way to a man's heart is through his stomach" certainly holds true in more the its original intention. There are a lot of ways to protect your heart, starting with diet. By adopting a balanced eating plan, you can control your weight, raise your levels of "good" cholesterol, and lower your levels of "bad" cholesterol. Supplement with nutrients such as magnesium, chromium, vitamin E, carnitine, coenzyme Q_{10}, and a variety of herbs to strengthen your heart muscle and protect against harmful free radicals. Avoid taking in too much iron to prevent iron overload. And don't forget about those important EFAs. There's a lot that you can control here. Your health is in your hands.

Chapter 10 will guide you in starting an exercise program to help regulate your cholesterol levels, improve circulation, and make your heart stronger and more efficient.

7.

Enhancing Your Sex Life

You can be a sexual dynamo at any age—without Viagra. All you have to do is generate some excess energy—that is, energy in excess of what is required to maintain the vital functions of the body. Sexual energy is surplus energy. It can be abundant in the healthy male, regardless of age.

There is a definite correlation between good health and good sex. When we're healthy, we're in balance. Balance confers on us, among other things, vigor and vitality, as well as a properly functioning hormonal system. The result is normal, healthy functioning.

Not only is good health necessary for proper sexual functioning, but it seems that the reverse is also true: A fulfilling sex life enhances physical, as well as emotional health. According to Alexander Lowen, M.D., executive director of the International Institute for Bioenergetic Analysis in New York City, both men and women who are sexually satisfied are much less likely to develop heart disease. One study, involving 131 men, ages thirty-one to eighty-six who had been hospitalized for heart attack, found that two-thirds reported suffering from sexual difficulties just prior to their heart attacks.

Sex is therapeutic for us. It helps relieve stress. By doing so, it may also enhance the body's immune function. The stress response involves a reduction in T-cell count and beta endorphin levels. T-cells are immune cells that fight off invading germs or other foreign bodies. Endorphins are brain chemicals that help us tune out pain. They're produced in large numbers during strenuous exercise and during sex. When stress is reduced, endorphin and T-cell production increase. Therefore, by alleviating stress, sexual activity can enhance immunity and reduce pain. The increased endorphin production that results from sexual activity may explain why it tends to relieve back pain and arthritis. In addition to blocking pain, endorphins also produce feelings of euphoria and exhilaration.

Nutritional deficiencies can leave you feeling fatigued, listless and depressed, with little—if any—energy left for sexual activity. Our bodies were not designed to handle chronic stress. While we can handle acute episodes of stress and recover, the increased stresses that today's man is under in our fast-paced, competitive society leave many continually exhausted. Nutritional needs sky-rocket during stressful periods. When these needs go unmet, additional stress is placed upon the body. As the nutritional gap widens, energy and stamina diminish. When we talk about restoring or enhancing sexual functioning, we're really talking about bringing energy and vitality back into the body, which is what getting healthy is all about.

Health is intimately linked with lifestyle and diet, and you are in control of these factors. You have the power to enhance your vitality and your sexuality. All you need is the right information on how nutritional and environmental factors affect sexual functioning. I will discuss effective and safe ways to deal with decreased sex drive, impotence, premature ejaculation, and infertility.

IMPOTENCE

An estimated 30 million American men suffer from impotence. Impotence literally means "no strength." It is a condition of erectile failure, where the male is either unable to get an adequate erection or unable to sustain it long enough to successfully complete intercourse.

According to J. Douglas Trapp, M.D., a board certified urologist and consultant to the Osborn Foundation Impotence Resource Center in Augusta, Georgia, about 15 percent of males everywhere are impotent. He claims that successful treatment is available for over 90 percent of the men so affected. Nonetheless, 60 percent of impotent men put off going to the doctor for at least a year.

A large advertisement run in a small town newspaper by a clinic specializing in treating impotency states that impotence is the "most common medical disorder in the world—almost as common as the cold, but much more treatable." It goes on to say that 95 percent of their patients are treated with medication. What it doesn't say is that a very large number of drugs can cause impotence. Among them are several classes of medication for hypertension, ulcers, and nausea, as well as seizure medications, antihistamines, sedatives, antidepressants, and tranquilizers. Use of cigarettes, alcohol, and street drugs can also be major causes of physical impotency.

It has been found that 90 percent of men with impotence are or have been heavy cigarette smokers. A study reported in 1994 in the *Journal of Epidemiology* involving 4,462 Vietnam veterans revealed that current smokers had 50 percent more reported impotence than non-smokers. So do you still need another reason to quit smoking?

Before 1980, the prevailing medical opinion about impotence had been that it was caused largely by psychological problems. However, the tides have turned, and today most cases of impotence are believed to stem from organic disorders. If a man is able to get an erection during sleep, masturbation, or sex with a different partner, organic causes can be ruled out and emotional causes should be assessed. The primary causes of psychological impotence are depression, marital problems, job stress, and performance anxiety. Immaturity and low self-esteem also can be contributing factors.

In addition to prescription and street drugs, alcohol, and cigarettes, impotency can be caused by any of the following physical factors:

- Cadmium toxicity.

- Circulatory insufficiency.

- Disorders of the nerves, such as multiple sclerosis or paralysis from an accident.

- Hormonal deficiency.

- Intense exercise.

- Radiation for pelvic cancer.

- Severe chronic diseases, such as cancer or cirrhosis of the liver.

- Severe kidney failure.

- Surgery.

Of these possible causes, intense exercise was found in a Michigan Medical Center study to lead to a drop in production of hormones involved in potency, fertility, and sex drive.

The next few pages discuss, in greater detail, two major factors that contribute to impotence: circulatory insufficiency and hormonal disorders.

Circulatory Insufficiency

Circulatory insufficiency is the most common cause of impotence in American men. Arteriosclerotic plaque on the walls of penile arteries can result in diminished blood supply to the penis. A study following the progress of 3,250 men, ages twenty-six to eighty-three found that high total cholesterol and low HDL tend to correlate with erectile dysfunction.[1] Clearly, keeping your arteries free of plaque is not only good for your heart, but it's good for your sexual performance as well.

Because of their ability to stimulate vascular flow to the penis, yohimbe and ginkgo biloba are two herbs that are often used to treat impotence caused by circulatory insufficiency. Ginkgo biloba extract was given to a group of men who were unresponsive to traditional drug therapy. In a six-month period, half of the group regained potency. One 40 milligram capsule taken daily can produce results in two months, though it may take up to six months to regain full potency.

I have many clients who absolutely swear by yohimbe. Its active ingredient, yohimbine, is derived from the African yohimbe tree. Yohimbine dilates surface blood vessels and stimulates the release of norepinephrine, which opens the vascular door to the penis. Yohimbine also decreases the latency period between ejaculations and has been demonstrated to increase libido. In a study done at Stanford University, three groups of rats (normal, virginal, and impotent) were injected with yohimbine. Afterwards, nearly half of the sexually inactive rats began copulating, while copulation in the normal group nearly doubled.

The usual dose of yohimbe bark standardized extract is one to two 50-milligram capsules daily. While yohimbine can increase heart rate and cause a slight increase in blood pressure, creating a feeling of nervousness, it is without serious side effects. Dr. Christian Barnard, pioneer in heart-transplant surgery, reports that three out of four heart transplant patients had immediate return of sexual potency after taking yohimbine.

> *George, a fifty-four-year-old architect, reluctantly came to see me at his wife's insistence. Six months earlier, he had undergone bypass surgery. After his convalescence, he was having a difficult time in the bedroom. He'd been following a moderate exercise program and really watching his diet. George had a notorious sweet tooth, but since his bypass, he had been careful with both sugar and bad fats.*
>
> *I started him on the Super Nutrition Sex Formula that included yohimbe bark standardized extract as well as other sexually supportive ingredients. I recommended one a day to start, and suggested he might want to take an additional one before an amorous evening. By the end of one week, George's wife called to tell me that the nutrients I had given him were beginning to work.*

The B vitamin niacin can also improve blood flow to the penis. It's a natural chelator. *Chelation* is a process in which certain nutrients bind with material obstructing the arteries and escort it out of the body. Natural chelators include vitamins B_6 and C, the minerals magnesium, manganese, and selenium, DMG (discussed later in this chapter), the enzyme bromelain, and the mineral salts orotic acid and aspartic acid.

The material that clogs arteries is made up largely of mineral deposits, laid down when minerals go out of solution as a consequence of pH imbalance. Since pH is regulated by electrolytes, they too can be viewed as chelating agents. In fact, electrolytes are known to be superior chelating agents. By correcting pH, they correct the basic conditions that give rise to the problem. Garlic, onions, and high-fiber foods also assist in the natural chelation process.

Hormonal Disorders

When one thinks of hormones in relation to impotence, testosterone is probably the first to come to mind. While testosterone is involved in sexual function, the pancreas, thyroid, and adrenal glands also produce hormones that affect human sexual functioning and response. In fact, diabetes causes 90 percent of hormonal impotence, and the hormone involved is, of course, insulin.

The adrenal glands, which produce the sex hormones, work together with the thyroid to produce and maintain the body's energy levels. And extra energy is what you're after for peak sexual performance. Our bodies were not designed to handle chronic stress. When the body experiences stress, the adrenal glands begin to hyperfunction. Once the stress is removed, the adrenals quiet down and return to their normal function. This is what the body was designed to do.

When stress continues, the adrenal glands draw energy from the body's nutrient reserves. When stress becomes a way of life, the body simply becomes exhausted. Reserves of energy and nutrition are totally depleted. Those who live with constant, unending worries about finances, family, health problems, and divorce, among other stresses, use up excessive amounts of nutritional

* For information on balanced hormonal therapy, write to Broda O. Barnes Research Foundation, P.O. Box 98 Trumbill, CT 06611, or call 203–261–2101.

reserves every day. And chances are if you're stressed out, you aren't eating right to begin with.

Stress to our physical bodies comes in many different forms. In addition to the emotional and mental stress we commonly think of, physical stress—including any physical injury, illness, overwork, or lack of sleep—affects the adrenals. Any chemical substance, whether from environmental pollutants or diets high in over-processed foods, refined sugar, and stimulants such as coffee, must be detoxified by the body. This puts stress on the adrenal glands. Lack of exercise or excessive exercise and the use of recreational drugs also contributes to burnout.

When the adrenals burn out, passion's flames are extinguished. If you're tired when you get up and spend the better part of your day spiking your overworked adrenal glands with caffeine, nicotine, sugar, and soda just to get through another day, there's not much energy left to spike you into sexual action in the evening.

Underproduction of thyroid hormones, known as *hypothyroidism,* can lead to many health disorders, among them fatigue and impotence. Again, the lack of energy necessary for peak sex performance and enjoyment is missing in a man suffering from hypothyroidism.

Testosterone deficiency interferes with erections and suppresses sexual desire. Testosterone levels decline with age. As they decline, so does sexual desire and performance, especially in men. It is testosterone that determines sex drive—in women, as well as men. At age twenty-five, the average free testosterone level in men is about 200 pg/ml. At age eighty, it's only about 10 pg/ml. As testosterone levels decrease with age, the incidence of impotence increases. The following statistics show percentages of impotence for each decade of life between ages forty and eighty:

age 40	2 percent
age 50	5 percent
age 60	18 percent
age 70	27 percent
age 80	75 percent

The figures above lend credence to the idea of "male menopause." Called andropause, its onset is more subtle than that of menopause in women, but it can nevertheless cause problems because of the symptoms it can produce. In addition to impotence, the symptoms of andropause include weakness, stiffness, pain, nervous exhaustion, loss of muscle tone, irritability, and profuse sweating, with intolerance to heat. According to William Campbell Douglass, M.D., "many of these problems will completely disappear with proper testosterone therapy."[2] In this case, "proper" means correct doses (small) of the correct form. For example, all men should avoid methyl-testosterone, because it damages the liver. The doses of testosterone used to counteract the symptoms of andropause are much smaller than those used by athletes who take steroids to increase muscle mass. In such large doses, testosterone can actually destroy the sex drive.*

One way to confirm the onset of andropause is by measuring levels of a hormone called *follicle-stimulating hormone* (FSH). It is a pituitary hormone that controls sex hormone secretion in both men and women. Andropause is heralded in by an increase in FSH levels, which can be measured in blood or urine collected over a twenty-four-hour period. Another way to verify onset of andropause is through the "estrogen urine test." Here the amount of male estrogen production is reflected in a day's output of urine. Amounts in excess of 20 micrograms indicate that the change has taken place.

TREATMENT OPTIONS FOR IMPOTENCE

Many men are likely to be told by their doctors that the only effective treatments for impotence involve implants, injections, or hormone therapy. These "cures" are often costly, and they do not address the underlying causes of the problem. The need for such medical treatments can be avoided, however, by making some simple lifestyle changes and supplementing with herbs and nutritional supplements. Let's take a look at the pros and cons of conventional medical treatment and herbal and nutrient therapies.

Conventional Medical Treatments

There are many devices available for men who are unable to achieve or sustain an erection because of a mechanical defect in the penis. These instruments produce an erection mechanically. For example, there is a condomlike device that works through a simple suction action. There are also vacuum devices available, in which a suction tube is placed over the penis to draw blood into it, and then a rubber constriction ring is applied, trapping the blood inside. The erection produced in this manner is somewhat unsteady, but it's sufficient to allow intercourse.

An alternative to these mechanisms is penile injection. In this case, the man injects a smooth muscle relaxant into the base of his penis, causing it to become engorged with blood. Depending upon the combination of drugs used and the dose, the erection can last from half an hour to an hour and a half. Although some men report quite satisfying results with this procedure, others find the method to be an unacceptable option.

A final alternative lies in surgical implants, in which a rod is inserted into the penis. There are three different models available, ranging from semi-rigid to completely inflatable. In one model, inflation and deflation is achieved by squeezing the scrotum. Implants have been in use since the 1970s. Increasingly good results are claimed by the medical profession, notwithstanding the wave of litigation a few years ago, resulting from improperly placed or defective devices.

The treatment of impotence is a growing medical specialty, and clinics generally offer mechanical devices, injections, and implants, as well as hormone therapy and vascular bypass surgery. Of these treatment options, hormone therapy may sound like the most acceptable; however, if the cause of the problem is vascular, rather than hormonal, it's of little benefit. While hormone therapy may seem a more natural approach than the others, keep in mind that hormonal output is largely determined by nutrient input. Balancing macronutrients, essential fatty acids, and electrolytes can do much to restore hormonal balance in the body, possibly eliminating the need for medical treatment with hormones.

Not counting the cost of diagnostic workup, the price of treatment in a medical clinic specializing in impotency can range from $500 per year for medication to more than $25,000 for surgery requiring a hospital stay. Impressive "cure" rates of 90 to 95 percent often refer to injection therapies that many men decline. Impotency clinics generally don't offer the less costly, less invasive nutritional therapies described in this chapter. As you will see, nutritional approaches come closer to offering a real cure, if we take the word to mean "correction of the underlying problem," rather than "relief of symptoms."

Nutritional Therapies

Super nutrition plays an important role in helping you handle stress, thereby enhancing your performance. While balanced nutrition won't solve your marital problems or eliminate common on-the-job pressures, it can optimize your ability to handle the stress of everyday living. Indeed, nutrition is probably your strongest ally when it comes to maximizing your manhood.

On the high-carbohydrate diet, the brain doesn't get its fair share of glucose, the only fuel it can use effectively. The glucose in the body is instead used as an energy source to run the rest of the body. The result is the development of hypoglycemic symptoms, many of which are emotional in nature. These can include fatigue, insomnia, headaches, nervous habits, and mental disturbances. Adopting the 40/30/30 eating plan and using unprocessed whole foods has a stabilizing effect on blood sugar, mood swings, attention span, focus, and long-term energy.

An intake of the right kinds of essential fatty acids helps the body produce prostaglandins, which you first learned about in Chapter 2. These help regulate sexual response. The gonads "make use of fatty acids for hormone production and for the transfer of neurogenital impulse waves to the brain."[3] Insufficient prostaglandins, due to lack of the omega-6 EFA gamma linoleic acid (GLA), can produce sexual dysfunctions such as insufficient ejaculate and infertility. Evening primrose oil and borage oil are excellent sources of GLA. They provide specific fatty acids that produce heightened sexual response. Spirulina is also rich in GLA, as well as being an excellent source of complete and highly digestible protein. It has been used to treat impotency, lack of libido, and premature ejaculation. And vitamin B_6 helps convert linoleic acid into prostaglandins.

For optimal sexual functioning, the thyroid and adrenal glands, as well as testicular function, must be supported nutritionally. Vitamin E and zinc nourish the sex glands, while adrenal support is provided by vitamins A, C, E, B complex (especially B_2 and pantothenic acid), and the EFAs. The thyroid gland is supported by iodine and the B vitamins, especially B_1 and pantothenic acid.

Remember that the proper balance of macronutrients produces "good" eicosanoids that regulate the cardiovascular system, and that circulatory insufficiency is the most common cause of impotence in our culture. American men can therefore protect their hearts *and* enhance their sexuality by adopting a balanced diet. Increasing your dietary intake of fish that are rich in the right fats may also help, as studies have shown that they increase blood levels of two omega-3 EFAs, EPA, and DHA. This may, in turn, help prevent cardiovascular problems and enhance sexual activity.

Vitamins and Minerals

Some of your most powerful weapons against impotence are vitamins and minerals, including vitamins A, B complex, C, and E, and manganese, phosphorus, selenium, and zinc. These beneficial nutrients work in a variety of ways to help improve sexual function. Some are stimulants, others are vital to testosterone production, and still others are important for thyroid and adrenal support. Whatever their functions, you should make sure that you're taking in adequate amounts of each of the following vitamins and minerals.

Vitamin A: Testicular tissue is maintained, in part, by vitamin A. Excellent sources of vitamin A include dairy products, eggs, fish liver oil, and yellow fruits and vegetables.

Vitamin B Complex: The B vitamins influence the production of testosterone. Vitamins B_1 and B_2 help support the thyroid and adrenal glands respectively. Together, these glands produce 98 percent of the body's energy. Pantothenic acid also supports the thyroid and the adrenals. When these glands are underactive, fatigue and diminished sex drive can result. Folic acid works in conjunction with testosterone to develop mature sperm. And another B complex vitamin, para-aminobenzoic acid (PABA), has been successfully used in the treatment of Peyronie's disease, a condition characterized by extreme curvature of the penis that makes erection quite painful. The best food sources for the B complex vitamins are brewer's yeast, liver, and whole-grain cereals.

Vitamin C: As a man ages, vitamin C becomes increasingly important to the proper functioning of his sex glands. If an insufficient amount is obtained from the diet, the sex glands will steal it from other body tissues. If there is none to steal, sex drive will diminish or vanish, as sex-gland function drops or stops altogether. Food rich in vitamin C include acerola cherries, broccoli, cantaloupe, citrus fruits, green peppers, rose hips, sprouted alfalfa seeds, and strawberries.

Vitamin E: Commonly known as the "sex vitamin," vitamin E works as an antioxidant. When the penis is erect, it is engorged with oxygen-rich blood. Vitamin E assists in transporting that oxygen and prevents its oxidation.

Good food sources of vitamin E include almonds, peanuts, cold-pressed oils, desiccated liver, eggs, leafy vegetables, organ meats, sweet potatoes, and wheat germ.

Manganese: Men who are impotent are commonly deficient in this essential trace mineral. Deficiency can generally be determined through hair analysis. Nuts, seeds, and whole-grain cereals are rich in manganese.

Phosphorus: This was the first mineral recognized as being directly involved with sex drive. Phosphorus is found in curries, chutneys, and hot sauces, all of which provide stimulation, in the form of irritation, to the sex organs. Underground fungi known as truffles contain phosphorus, and these are purported to have an aphrodisiac effect. Phosphorus is also present in lecithin in the form of phospholipids, a combination of nitrogen, fatty acids, and glycerol, that promote sex-hormone secretion. Lecithin can be produced in the body only in the presence of the B vitamins—especially B_6.

Good food sources of phosphorus include brewer's yeast, pumpkin, squash, sunflower seeds, and wheat bran and germ.

Selenium: Nearly half of the selenium in a man's body can be found in his testicles and in portions of the seminal ducts alongside the prostate gland. Since selenium is scarce in our food supply and vital to proper sexual functioning, men need to make sure that they take in plenty of this important trace mineral. Foods high in selenium include Brazil nuts, brewer's yeast, butter, herring, sesame seeds, tuna, wheat germ and bran, and whole grains.

Zinc: This mineral is vital to the production of testosterone, and a deficiency can result in impotence and reduced sperm count. Zinc helps guard against cadmium toxicity, which can result in impotence. Cadmium toxicity is common among smokers. A man's ability to absorb zinc declines with age, and the mineral is destroyed by drugs, alcohol, coffee, and smoking, as well as by infections.

Brewer's yeast, eggs, herring, meats, mushrooms, organ meats, pumpkin and sunflower seeds, seafood (especially oysters), soybeans, and wheat germs are all rich dietary sources of zinc.

Herbal Treatments

Herbs seem to work best if taken in cycles, rather than on a continuous basis. This way the body remains more responsive to their effects. For maximum benefit, you may wish to alternate the herbs and herbal combinations that you take.

Ginseng: This popular and effective herb helps the body to overcome stress and fatigue and to regain strength. Ginseng does this by supporting the adrenals. There are many varieties of this herb available, including Korean, Chinese, Siberian, and American. The Manchurian variety from China is particularly helpful in rejuvenating the male reproductive system, because it stimulates the endocrine glands to increase testosterone production.

Ginseng has been studied extensively. Laboratory tests with mice and rats showed that following an injection with a ginseng extract, the animals copulated more frequently. Increased growth of organs, especially the gonads, was also noted. As a stimulant, ginseng may produce side effects such as insomnia, irritability, and nervousness, especially if taken over a long period of time.

Sarsaparilla: This herb is rich in plant steroids known as phytosterols. Sarsaparilla nourishes sex hormones and can therefore be useful in treating impotence.

Saw Palmetto: The saw palmetto tree (*Serenoa repens*) is indigenous to the southeastern states of North America. The tree has grape-sized berries that range in color from reddish black to brown in color. Extracts from these berries, called liposterolic extracts, are beneficial in treating disorders of the prostate gland, as you first learned in Chapter 5. As it turns out, saw palmetto can also be useful in treating impotence. It not only help to build strength, but is considered by some to be an aphrodisiac.

True unicorn root: Reported to be an excellent herbal medicine for impotence, true unicorn root has also been used to promote fertility in both sexes.

Lack of iodine and the amino acid phenylalanine, which breaks down into tyrosine (see page 131), can cause a decrease of thyroid hormones. Bayberry, black cohosh, and goldenseal can help support thyroid function. Because of their high mineral content, sea vegetables are also beneficial. Zinc, manganese, and the B vitamins are needed for healthy thyroid function, as well.

Other herbs that support the adrenal glands include licorice root, hops, passionflower, and skullcap. Stress exhausts these glands and depletes the body of vital minerals including calcium, magnesium, zinc, potassium, sodium, and copper. Eating sea vegetables, such as dulse, hijiki, arame, and nori, is an excellent way to replace these minerals and improve the health of the adrenals. The B complex vitamins and vitamin C are also vital in supporting and maintaining adrenal function.

Other Nutrients

There are a variety of natural food supplements and amino acids that can be beneficial for men who are impotent. These include aloe vera juice; the amino acids dimethylglycine and tyrosine; bee pollen and honey; and Royal jelly.

Aloe vera juice: Due to the properties of its oils, vitamins, minerals, and amino acids, aloe vera juice is said to have sexually stimulating properties. It's also very healing for internal organs. One half cup of the clear gel, taken daily, is recommended for this purpose.

Dimethylglycine (DMG): An over-the-counter food compound, once known as pangamic acid or vitamin B_{15}, DMG is an amino acid that "acts as a cofactor, aiding vitamins, fats, hormones, and proteins in completing their metabolic action or cycle."[4] DMG aids in detoxifying the body by increasing oxygen utilization at the cellular level. This results in increased muscle tone of the organs, including the sexual organs, and restores the elasticity and strength of the penis.

DMG also helps combat fatigue at doses of one or two 90-milligram tablets daily. It improves circulation and normalizes blood levels of several hormones by stimulating the adrenal glands, which are important to sexual functioning. Additionally, DMG increases cellular production of lecithin, which is found in high amounts in male reproductive fluid and helps promote sex hormone secretion.

Tyrosine: People with low levels of the brain chemicals norepinephrine and adrenaline, which control mood, sex drive, and energy level, are more prone to depression and loss of libido. The amino acid tyrosine is directly involved in the production of these chemicals. Tyrosine is also a precursor to another neurotransmitter called dopamine, which is also involved with sexual drive.

There is evidence that small doses of tyrosine are more effective in increasing brain levels of neurotransmitters than are large doses. Doses of 1,000 milligrams, taken in the morning and at night, can be administered when blood levels are low, with a gradual increase to 2,000 milligrams twice a day. Tyrosine has also been shown to lower blood pressure and suppress appetite. Supplemental tyrosine is not recommended for anyone who has the skin cancer melanoma, or for individuals taking MAO inhibitors—certain drugs used in the treatment of depression. In addition, women who are pregnant should not supplement with tyrosine.

In addition to the nutrients listed above, there are several other supplements that can help improve sexual function. Bees produce three substances that are believed to have sexual benefits for men. One of these, pollen, contains natural hormonal substances that stimulate and nourish the reproductive system and help increase sexual stamina. Another product, which is known as Royal jelly, can be of benefit for impotence and sterility. And honey, too, increases potency, as well as the body's production of sex hormones. However, remember to go easy with such concentrated sweet substances, because they can create havoc with blood-sugar levels by triggering the insulin response.

INFERTILITY

It's considered somewhat normal for fertility to decline with age. Sperm production normally decreases by more than half as men age from twenty to eighty. However, infertility is *not* normal and is a sign of a depleted system. Infertility affects approximately 15 percent of all couples. Those unable to conceive generally want to be tested to get to the root of the problem. They are usually advised to wait at least at a year before doing so, as conception occurs among 80 percent of fertile couples after one year of trying. One-third of infertility is a result of female sterility, one-third results from male sterility, and the other one-third stems from the combined conditions of both partners. Although men are no more often the source of the problem than women, it's recommended that they be tested first because the procedures involved are simpler. Understand, however, that infertility screening is costly and often unproductive. Medicine is able to find the sources of infertility in only 60 percent of the men tested.

Before embarking upon screening, couples may want to work on correcting lifestyle habits such as smoking and drinking, modifying stress, and taking nutritional supplements to help protect genetic material in the sperm and ova. Couples unable to conceive may also want to test the advice of medical experts: Have intercourse every other night from day ten to day eighteen of the menstrual cycle and avoid the use of lubricants. Women should not douche after having intercourse.

The average man today produces only half as much sperm as his grandfather did. A study conducted in 1992 found that sperm counts among men in industrialized nations declined 50 percent in a fifty-year period. These findings are consistent with more recent studies published in the *New England Journal of Medicine* and the *British Medical Journal.* They report a decline in sperm count between 33 and 41 percent in recent years.

Male infertility can be caused by congenital defects, including the absence of the spermatic duct or testes that did not descend properly; hormonal imbalance; "street" and prescription drugs; chemicals; radiation; infections; the existence of sperm antibodies; varicocele (a varicose vein draining a testis); and retrograde ejaculation, a common result of prostate surgery (see Chapter 5). Men who wear tight jeans are more likely to develop problems with fertility. This may be due to restricted circulation to the genitals that can lead to reduced sperm count. And, in addition to possibly increasing the risk of heart disease, iron overload can cause infertility and impotence. Men suffering from these conditions may want to rule out hereditary hemochromatosis through the laboratory tests, as discussed in Chapter 6. Finally, while hot tubs and saunas are often used for relaxation and to enhance sexual encounters, they can also result in reduced sperm counts.

It seems that a major cause of decreased sperm production among men almost everywhere in the "civilized" world is the widespread use of industrial and agricultural chemicals such as Dioxin. These are chemically similar to estrogen and have a toxic effect upon the body by acting like estrogen in the body. When pregnant women are exposed to these hormone-mimicking chemicals, their male offspring are born with fewer sperm-producing sertoli cells. Increasing numbers of reproductive-tract abnormalities have resulted from exposure to these chemicals in our food, air, and water.

Nutritional Therapies

Even when sperm count is normal, reduced motility, or swimming ability, can contribute to infertility. Where both are present—low sperm count coupled with lowered motility—a man's chances of being infertile are greatly increased. Researchers have discovered that both motility and fertility of sperm are proportionate to the amount of vitamin E in the semen. Experiments on rats have shown that when a group was fed a diet adequate in all other respects, but lacking in vitamin E, the first generation of rats became partially sterile, the second generation completely sterile. Vitamin E is an important antioxidant nutrient that is largely lacking in processed foods—which are *not* lacking in the typical American diet. I recommend supplementation with 400 to 600 international units daily in the form of mixed tocopherols. Selenium, as the mineral activator of the vitamin E complex, is also needed. Try supplementing with 300 micrograms per day.

Vitamin A is also important to fertility. It promotes the formation of a higher number of sperm in the ejaculate. Vitamins C, vitamin E, and the B vitamin folic acid, as well as the essential fatty acids, are all important for healthy sperm production.

Vitamin B_{12} has been successfully used in treating male sterility. This nutrient, plus the B vitamin inositol, vitamin C, and the minerals calcium, magnesium, zinc, and sulfur, are all found in healthy sperm and so may be necessary for fertility.

Another nutrient that benefits both sperm count and motility is carnitine. Once considered an amino acid, carnitine is now classified as an amine—a nitrogen-containing compound. In a recent study, a dose of 3 grams of carnitine was given daily to 100 infertile men with sperm motility problems.[5] At the end of four months, increased sperm motility and sperm count were noted, with the most dramatic improvements occurring in those men who entered the study with the poorest sperm motility.

The essential amino acid arginine can also be useful in doses of up to eight grams. In 80 percent of men with low counts, 4 grams per day can increase sperm count. However, arginine is not recommended in doses exceeding 30 milligrams for men with a history of schizophrenia, because it can aggravate symptoms through its chemical action. Arginine is also contraindicated in cases of herpes simplex infection. Men with this condition should avoid arginine-rich foods—primarily nuts and seeds—as well. They may also want to consider supplementing their diet with lysine.

Studies have shown that if more than 20 percent of sperm are clumped together, termed *sperm agglutination,* conception cannot take place. In one study, men given 500 milligrams of vitamin C every twelve hours showed an 11 percent decrease in sperm agglutination after three weeks. Vitamin C is important in guarding against sperm damage that can cause birth defects and childhood illnesses.

Histamine is a chemical in our cells and blood that controls ejaculation. The family of B vitamins, especially niacin and folic acid, as well as fatty acids, can help in some cases of infertility, for they raise blood histamine levels. Men too low in histamine can't achieve ejaculation. Inversely, men with high levels of histamine, may ejaculate prematurely.

PREMATURE EJACULATION

In order to determine if an ejaculation is premature or timely, we need some guideline as to how much time it normally takes for a man to ejaculate. It might surprise you to learn that, in the average sexual encounter, only three minutes elapse from the man's first thought of having sex until the act culminates in ejaculation. For a woman, the average time between arousal and orgasm is thirteen minutes.

Doctors have sometimes prescribed circumcision for premature ejaculation because it decreases the sensitivity of the penis. However, the majority of men in our society are already circumcised. So it may be helpful for men to wear a condom—or two or three—during intercourse to avoid overstimulation that may lead to premature ejaculation. Some men choose to masturbate before having intercourse. The reasoning here is that subsequent erections will last longer.

It can also be helpful for men to learn to control the sensations that lead up to ejaculation. One technique for this is to practice delaying ejaculation during extended foreplay. The partner squeezes the penis lightly when the man reports an approaching sensation of orgasm. An alternative is the "stop-start" technique that substitutes interrupted foreplay for squeezing when the male senses that ejaculation is forthcoming.

Doctors have found that physical disorders are rarely the cause of premature ejaculation. In some cases, however, premature ejaculation can be caused by high histamine levels. Elevated histamine is associated with allergies. Men with allergies therefore may tend to ejaculate sooner than men without them. Supplementing with calcium and the amino acid methionine can help lower blood histamine.

ENHANCING THE ENCOUNTER

Aphrodisiacs, named after Aphrodite, the Greek goddess of love, beauty, and fruitfulness, are substances that increase sexual arousal. Through the ages, about 2,000 substances have been purported to have aphrodisiac effects. Dr. Morton Walker tells us that "the physiological basis for some aphrodisiacal claims is that when the substance is eaten, drunk or rubbed on the body, it acts on nerve centers in the brain to decrease inhibitions."[6]

According to the teachings of Eastern medicine, the kidneys govern sexual vitality. Excessive intake of coffee, alcohol, fatty foods, or emotional stress can irritate the kidneys, while warmth nourishes these organs—and therefore sexual energy. Along these lines, eating too many cold foods, such as fruits and salads, or drinking iced beverages—especially in cold weather—can "cool one's passion."

To warm the kidneys and nourish sexual energy, you need to eat foods like beans; whole grains; green, leafy vegetables; and seeds. Seeds not only contain the germ of life, but they are an excellent source of zinc, which is found in abundance in seminal fluid. Oysters, also rich in zinc, are said to have been the "love tonic" of Casanova. Organic fertile eggs have also been considered to have aphrodisiac properties, and so have garlic, artichokes, mushrooms, and caviar. Fish have been long thought to stimulate sexual activity and, for that reason, priests were at one time forbidden to eat them. Many of the culinary spices, because of their warming and gentle, stimulating nature are also considered to be aphrodisiacs. These include ginger, cloves, cardamom, anise, caraway, nutmeg, vanilla, and cinnamon.

Aphrodisiacs can also include substances applied externally to the genitals. Medicine has employed the use of nitroglycerine paste applied directly to the penis to help impotence. (It does not have this effect when taken orally, though.) Musk oil, from the musk ox, has traces of sheep testosterone in it, and ambergris is a gray, waxy substance excreted in the intestines of sperm whales. Either of these oils may be rubbed into the penis (after it has been washed and dried) one hour prior to intercourse to enhance the experience. These oils "cause a contractile reaction in the muscles of the penis, so erectile tissues can remain stiff."[7] They can also be applied to the clitoris.

Musk and ambergris also have a pleasant scent. Women react most to musk-like smells. Men and women both can become sexually stimulated through the olfactory sense, it seems, in subconscious reaction to chemicals called *pheromones*. Most animals and humans secrete these chemicals as a component of perspiration. About 10 percent of men secrete a pheromone called androsterone in their perspiration. It has been proven that women find these men exceptionally appealing, being aroused subconsciously by the pheromones they sense.

Actually, androsterone is produced in the adrenal glands of both sexes, so women secrete this pheromone, too. And it's also found in the vaginal labia and in the foreskin of the penis. In the 1970s, an aerosol spray called Bodywise, containing androsterone, came to the United States from Great Britain. Theoretically, such a product could help correct sexual dysfunction.

The sense of smell can be further stimulated by the use of essential oils. Aphrodisiac oils include Jasmine, ylang-ylang, cinnamon, aniseed, clove buds, ginger root, nutmeg, peppermint, pepper, and rose. A few drops of these oils can be placed onto the mattress. To further enhance the atmosphere, orange, magenta, and purple decor are said to increase arousal. Candle light, soft music, and flowers—the old standbys—can help, too.

During orgasm, both men and women experience a sexual flush as a result of histamine release in the body. The B vitamin niacin produces a similar flush. It also increases sexual lubrication, by stimulating activity in the mucus membranes of the mouth and vagina. Taking 50 to 150 milligrams of niacin fifteen to thirty minutes prior to a sexual encounter can enhance the sexual flush and mucus membrane activity.

SUMMING IT UP

While a healthy body is necessary for proper sexual functioning, a satisfying sex life can, in turn, enhance your emotional and physical health. However, the stresses of daily life all too often take their toll, causing the adrenals to become exhausted and leading to such problems as fatigue, depression, decreased immunity, and hormonal imbalance—common causes of impotence. Circulatory insufficiency can also cause or contribute to impotence. If this is the case, you may find herbs that improve circulation, including yohimbe and ginkgo biloba, to be extremely helpful in restoring normal sexual functioning. Traditional herbal therapies, along with nutritional support in the form of vitamin B_6, vitamin C, magnesium, manganese, selenium, and a variety of other nutrients can help you enhance your sex life without having to rely on conventional medical treatments.

Infertility in males may be caused by birth defects and restricted circulation, in addition to the same problems of hormonal imbalance and the use of "street" or prescription drugs. And research shows that sperm counts have declined dramatically over the last fifty years due to environmental toxins—namely, the widespread use of industrial and agricultural chemicals. Evidence now suggests that vitamin E greatly affects the motility and fertility of sperm. Vitamin A, vitamin B complex, vitamin C, and inositol have been found in healthy sperm, and so are likely to be important for healthy sperm production. The same goes for the minerals calcium, magnesium, sulfur, and zinc. Promising studies have also shown carnitine to be beneficial for men with poor sperm motility.

Adrenal and thyroid support, along with a strong immune system, are vital to restoring sexual energy. Again, I can't stress enough the importance of balance in achieving and maintaining optimal health. When you attain balance in your diet and lifestyle, you restore your body's homeostasis, which ultimately leads to a positive attitude, a healthy body, and a satisfying sex life.

8.

Minimizing Hair Loss

You already know that Super Nutrition can make a big difference in many areas of your life. And, believe it or not, balanced nutrition really can help slow or stop the progression of hair loss. You can keep a full head of hair when you know the right steps to take. In fact, even if thinning has set in, there's a lot you can do to minimize further loss. Research is continuously shedding new light on the causes of hair loss in men, leading to the development of effective new treatments. Armed with a nutritional arsenal, you *can* prevent or reverse hair loss.

An estimated 30 million men experience loss or thinning of their hair as they age. About the same number are affected by impotence. Though the two are not related, what they have in common is that hormonal factors feature heavily in their cause. In this chapter, we'll look at these and other causes of hair loss in men and explore some nutritional, medical, and other approaches to minimizing the problem.

COMMON TYPES OF HAIR LOSS

Hairs fall out and are replaced by new ones on a regular basis. Loss of 50 to 100 hairs per day is normal. But problems result when lost hairs aren't replaced right away, aren't replaced at all, or are replaced with inferior quality hair.

There are three phases of hair growth: the anagen, catagen, and telogen phases. The anagen phase is the growing phase, normally lasting two to six years. The catagen phase is a transitional one that should last only about three weeks. Hairs that have entered the telogen, or resting phase, remain dormant in the scalp for two to four months, and then are pushed out by a new hair growing in the same root. In men with hair loss problems, however, the telogen phase is extended, lasting for several years—or for the remainder of their lives.

MALE PATTERN BALDNESS

In the form of hair loss known as male pattern baldness (MPB), or alopecia hereditaria, normal hairs called *terminal hairs* are replaced by fine, nearly invisible *vellus hairs*. Over the years, more and more terminal hairs are replaced by these barely visible vellus hairs, as the hair root decreases in size. As a result, a man with this type of thinning hair may appear to be bald. This is not the case, however, because in true baldness, the roots of the hair have withered and the hair follicles have died.

Male pattern baldness accounts for about 90 percent of hair loss cases. It affects approximately half of all males in Western industrialized countries. MPB is a form of *androgenetic hair loss*, meaning that it is caused by genes and male hormones. This kind of hair loss is believed to be caused by a "baldness gene" that is passed down by one parent. Dihydrotestosterone (DHT), a metabolite of testosterone, is also thought to be a primary factor in shrinking hair follicles and subsequent hair loss. As we discussed in Chapter 5, DHT levels increase with age, and this increase has been associated with prostate problems. That hormones are somehow involved with hair loss in males is certain because castrated men never lose their hair. But castration is obviously too extreme an alternative to prevent hair loss!

Male pattern baldness first shows up as a receding hair line that can manifest at a very early age—sometimes shortly after a man has reached sexual maturity. It has been found that balding men are deficient in the enzyme aromatase. When this enzyme is present in sufficient quantity, follicles grow hair. When there's not enough aromatase, follicles "turn off," stopping hair growth. The pattern in MPB is that hair loss is confined to the top of the head, although we still do not know why it's limited to this particular area.

Alopecia hereditaria (MPB) is just one of about three dozen different types of alopecia, all characterized by partial or total hair loss. Alopecia universalis is loss of hair all over the body. Alopecia areata is a sudden loss of hair in patches on the head, beard, and other parts of the body.

COMMON CAUSES OF HAIR LOSS

Among the possible causes of the various types of hair loss are:

- Acute illness
- Diabetes
- Drugs
- Excessive vitamin A intake
- Heavy metal toxicity
- High fever
- Iron deficiency
- Parasites
- Poor circulation
- Poor diet
- Radiation
- Skin disease
- Stress
- Sudden weight loss
- Thyroid disease
- Tight connective tissue in scalp
- Trauma
- Vitamin deficiency

Drugs that can cause hair loss include chemotherapeutic agents; antibiotics, including penicillin, sulfonamides, and mycin; heparin, an anticoagulant, or blood thinner; and carbimazole, a drug for the treatment of hyperthyroidism.

While poor circulation may contribute to hair loss, it is not a necessary and sufficient condition to cause the problem on its own.

If it were, stroke victims would lose their hair, hair transplants wouldn't work, and bald men wouldn't bleed when cut on the scalp. Nevertheless, activities aimed at improving circulation—massage, exercise, and the use of a slant board for fifteen minutes per day—can be useful adjunctive therapies when paired with other corrective measures. It may be worth it to try some of these possible therapies to see if you have any positive results.

UNSUSPECTED CAUSES OF HAIR LOSS

In addition to the factors listed on page 143, there are several causes of hair loss that doctors overlook. These include B-vitamin deficiencies, hypothyroidism, and parasites. If you have eliminated other possible causes of hair loss, you may want to be examined by a health-care professional to see if any of the following problems are involved.

Nutritional Deficiencies

Vitamin deficiencies that can lead to hair loss include insufficient inositol and para-aminobenzoic acid (PABA). These B vitamins protect hair follicles. When animals are put on a diet lacking inositol, their hair falls out. When it's added to the diet, their hair grows back. Hair loss for male animals is twice that of females, indicating a greater need for inositol among males. Also, a deficiency of the B vitamin biotin can cause hair loss.

PABA not only protects hair follicles, it has also been found effective in restoring natural hair color. When deprived of this vitamin, the hair of laboratory animals turns gray. Prematurely graying hair can also be caused by a deficiency of the amino acid phenylalanine, which is enzymatically related to melanin, the hair color pigment. Biotin, folic acid, and pantothenic acid can be helpful in restoring hair color, as well. My male clients absolutely swear by a special biotin product that Uni-Key (1–800–888–4353) now carries.

For your hair's sake, it's also vitally important to supply your body with nutrients that will support the thyroid gland. If the thyroid is underactive—and almost 40 percent of Americans are walking around with underactive thyroids—this can lead to hair loss. Hypothyroidism is a major factor in hair loss that should not be overlooked.

Hypothyroidism

Hypothyroidism, the underproduction of the hormones of the thyroid gland, is the underlying cause of many recurring illnesses. The condition may be hereditary or it may result from an iodine deficiency. According to Hal Huggins, D.D.S., there is also evidence that hypothyroidism is connected to silver/mercury dental amalgams. In the elderly, the condition is often mistaken for senility.

Hypothyroidism is characterized by the following symptoms:

- Constipation
- Dry, scaly skin
- Dull, dry hair
- Fatigue
- Hair loss
- Impaired intellectual capacity
- Impotence
- Loss of appetite
- Low sperm count
- Myxedema (drooping, swollen eyes)
- Night blindness
- Numbness, tingling in extremities
- Recurrent infections
- Sensitivity to cold
- Slurred speech

Iodine is an element with a very high specific gravity. The higher the specific gravity of an element, the stronger the gastric juices must be in order to extract and assimilate the element. The strength of gastric juice is reflected in pH, which, as you remember, is regulated by electrolytes. Without the trace minerals needed for electrolyte formation, pH balance is upset and gastric secretions are not strong enough to utilize iodine, even when it is supplied amply in the diet. Clearly, then, it's not enough to include more iodine in your diet—you also need to take in the electrolytes that are so important to proper thyroid function.

Sea vegetables are good for your hair and for healthy thyroid function. Kelp and dulse are both excellent sources of organic iodine, and all sea vegetables are rich sources of other trace minerals that help keep your electrolytes sparking.

A simple way to test yourself for an underactive thyroid gland is to take your armpit temperature first thing in the morning. This method was developed by Broda Barnes, M.D., a heart specialist and endocrinologist. Place a shake-down-type thermometer next to your bed before retiring. Upon awakening, and before rising, place it under your arm and lie still for fifteen minutes. A reading under 97.6°F may indicate of hypothyroidism. Repeat the procedure on several mornings and take an average of the readings. If it is 97°F or less you may want to consider taking a raw thyroid glandular. Armour thyroid is recommended, although it's available only with a prescription.

Treating Hypothyroidism

The amino acids tyrosine and phenylalanine can be useful in treating hypothyroidism. Tyrosine is a precursor of thyroid hormones. It is derived from phenylalanine, which is also a precursor of several neurotransmitters, including dopamine, norepinephrine, and epinephrine. Take up to three 500-milligram capsules of phenylalanine daily, or supplement with tyrosine, four to ten capsules taken daily in two or three equal doses. Make sure you take your tyrosine on an empty stomach.

The family of B vitamins improves cellular oxygenation and energy. These nutrients are extremely important for proper thyroid function. Because not all of the B vitamins in the naturally occurring compound have been synthesized, I recommend adding foods that are rich in these vitamins to the diet, in addition to taking a B complex supplement. Brewer's yeast and whole grains are excellent sources of the B vitamins.

If you have hypothyroidism, it's imperative that you avoid fluoride and chlorine because they block iodine receptors in the thyroid gland. Purifying drinking water through reverse osmosis or distillation will remove both fluoride and chlorine. However, when you drink water that's purified or distilled, remember to replenish the minerals using a liquid electrolyte formula such Trace-Lyte (see Chapter 3).

Certain foods contain a chemical known as goitrogen that blocks iodine absorption by the thyroid gland. These foods include:

- Broccoli
- Brussels sprouts
- Cabbage
- Cauliflower
- Kale
- Peanuts
- Rutabaga
- Soybeans
- Turnips
- Watercress

Cooking foods inactivates goitrogen, but you should still be careful to eat the foods listed above only in moderation. Your diet must also contain adequate protein, because a protein deficiency can inhibit thyroid activity.

Be aware that sulfa drugs and antihistamines can depress thyroid function and so should be used only under a doctor's order.

Parasites

Parasites are not well recognized as a cause of hair loss. Medical texts list diarrhea and malabsorption as symptoms of parasitic infection. But it doesn't end there. The fact is, any degenerative disease can be associated with parasites because they create a mucous overlay in the gut that blocks absorption, so we're unable to fully utilize the nutrients we take in.

Progressive, contemporary researchers are finding that parasites can cause a wide array of problems that include:

- Allergies
- Anemia
- Constipation
- Irritability/nervousness
- Joint pain
- Muscle cramps

- Digestive complaints
- Disturbed sleep
- Gas, bloating
- Irritable bowel syndrome

- Overall fatigue
- Persistent skin problems
- Post-nasal drip
- Teeth grinding

Parasites can contribute to hair loss because of their immuno-suppressive effect. Any man experiencing hair loss who also has one or more of the above symptoms and has ruled out other causes of hair loss may want to investigate the possibility of parasitic infection.

Many Americans erroneously believe that parasites are only a problem for people who travel to exotic places. But parasites are a here-and-now problem. This fact was brought home in a research paper that appeared in June 1994 in *The American Journal of Tropical Medicine and Hygiene.* The paper summarized findings from a study conducted by the Center for Disease Control and Prevention in Atlanta, Georgia, which showed that in 1987, and again in 1991, stool examinations by state diagnostic laboratories revealed parasites in 20 percent of all samples.

Among the most common of the microscopic organisms found in the study were *Giardia lamblia, Entamoeba coli,* and *Entamoeba histolytica.* Since these parasites were identified using standard stool analysis techniques, we may assume that the actual incidence of parasitic infection is even greater than the study suggests, for there is a 60-percent chance of missing parasites even when three consecutive standard stool analyses are performed. It takes more specialized testing techniques to reduce the number of false negative results. Even then, there is still a good chance of error. Parasites tend to hide in the lining (lumen) of the intestines, and they live in other organs and in the blood, as well.

The problem of parasites started making the headlines in the 1990s in connection with the Desert Storm veterans. They came to our attention again in 1993, when the microscopic organism, *Crytosporidium,* found its way into the city water supply in Milwaukee, Wisconsin. Four hundred thousand people developed stomach ailments and diarrhea, and 104 people died. The following year, the presence of the same organism in New York City's water supply was documented on NBC's television show, *Dateline*.

According to the Environmental Protection Agency (EPA), *Cryptosporidium* is currently the leading cause of waterborne illness in the United States, appearing in 80 percent of our surface water and 28 percent of drinking water samples. It poses a serious threat, especially to individuals with immunosuppressive disorders who can die from exposure to just a few of these organisms. Another prevalent water-borne parasite is *Giardia lamblia*. Chlorination does not kill either of these organisms. However, in November 1994, the EPA required all urban water systems to test for both *Crystosporidium* and *Giardia lamblia*.

Parasites can be brought to our shores by international travelers and immigrants. They can spread through restaurants where immigrants are frequently employed in food preparation, and day-care centers where workers come in contact with contaminated feces. Some parasites are sexually transmitted, some are passed on to us by our pets, and others are carried by "vectors" such as mosquitoes.

Preventing and Treating Parasitic Infection

The problem of parasitic infection is much more widespread than we've suspected. Most physicians don't expect to find parasites and therefore don't look for them. Even if they did, parasites are hard to find. The problem, therefore, tends to be underdiagnosed—and also misdiagnosed, since parasite symptoms tend to mimic other diseases. To rule out parasitic infection, you'll want to find a doctor who uses a lab that does either the purged stool analysis or the mucosal swab test, as these are more reliable than the standard stool analysis.* If the problem is correctly diagnosed, it's often treated with drugs such as Flagyl, Vermox, Iodiquinol, and Atabrine. These may cause side effects that include nausea, mental disturbances, and liver problems.

---

* If you have trouble locating a parasite specialist, you can call Uni-Key Health Systems at 1-800-888-4353 to order a state-of-the-art parasite test kit that has been made available to my readers and clients through an association between my office, Uni-Key, and a certified parasite laboratory. You can perform the test at home and the results can be quite helpful in detecting this difficult-to-diagnose condition.

Alternative treatments make use of herbs—black walnut, butternut, Ficus, garlic, mugwort, pink root, and wormwood—to fight larger parasites. Smaller organisms can be eliminated with grapefruit seed extract and enzymes like protease, papain, and bromelain, which break through their mucous overlay. These herbs may be taken alone or in combination with herbal laxatives such as senna or cascara sagrada. Generally, capsules or tinctures are taken three times a day for about two weeks, followed by a rest period of about five days. The cycle is then repeated once or twice more, depending upon symptoms.

The key to keeping parasite-free is to build a strong immune system. We can't do this without enough hydrochloric acid (HCl) in the stomach. HCl production tends to decline with age and is also low in people who eat a vegetarian diet. In addition, men with type A blood are genetically predisposed to achlorhydria, a condition in which the stomach does not produce enough hydrochloric acid. Two to four capsules or tablets of hydrochloric acid with meals can help correct the problem.

Stay away from sugar, including fruit sugar and especially refined sugar, because parasites are drawn to it as much as we are. And perhaps the most important thing you can do to eliminate or prevent parasites is to keep a clean colon that is well populated with beneficial, or "friendly," bacteria. Eating fiber-rich fruits, vegetables, and whole grains and taking lactobacillus supplements can help. It's also important to minimize your intake of substances that will destroy friendly bacteria. These include antibiotics, caffeine, fluoride, chlorine, mercury found in silver dental fillings, and refined carbohydrates.

TREATMENT OPTIONS FOR HAIR LOSS

Until recent years, the only suggestion that dermatologists had to offer to remedy hair loss was to avoid stress, get plenty of rest, and use medicated shampoo. Some doctors also recommended taking vitamins—usually a totally inadequate multivitamin. These days, drugs such as Rogaine are available for men who wish to minimize hair loss. While these drugs have been proven effective for some men, they don't offer a cure, in the true sense of the word—and they come with a long list of warnings and possible side effects. Fortunately, the right combination of nutrients can again come to the rescue to slow or stop the progression of hair loss. And there are some new approaches to treatment that have shown great promise in research studies.

Conventional Medical Treatment

In 1989, Upjohn Company received approval to market their minoxidil lotion, Rogaine, promising hope for many men who were concerned by their thinning hair. Minoxidil was not originally formulated to stimulate hair growth—it was widely prescribed by cardiologists for hypertension. According to Michael Oppenheim, M.D., "Around 1980, a number of formerly balding cardiologists became remarkably hairy."[1]

Minoxidil lotion is designed to be rubbed into the scalp. It stimulates new hair growth by blocking the action of testosterone on hair follicles, reversing their shrinkage. However, if they have shrunk too much, minoxidil won't work. For this reason, Dr. Oppenheim believes that the drug is best used as a preventative. He recommends that men start using it at age eighteen and take it for the rest of their lives! Twice a day applications produce noticeable results in six months unless the man is totally bald, in which case it may not work at all. The more hair on the scalp, the more will be generated as a result of using the lotion.

The problem with minoxidil is that new hair growth is apparently not limited to the head, but can spring up on the forehead, ears, and other places where hair is not supposed to grow. And hair growth is not the only side effect of minoxidil. In tablet form, the blood pressure medicine can cause salt and water retention, angina, rapid heart beat, and inflammation of the sac that surrounds the heart.

While it is unlikely that these symptoms will occur in men from use of the Rogaine lotion, it is possible—especially for men with heart disease. Rogaine may also have adverse effects when used in conjunction with blood pressure medications. According to the *Physician's Desk Reference Family Guide to Prescription Drugs,* the following side effects may occur from use of Rogaine for hair loss:

- Aches and pains
- Anxiety
- Arthritis symptoms
- Back pain
- Blood disorders
- Bone fractures
- Bronchitis
- Changes in blood pressure
- Changes in pulse rate
- Chest pain
- Conjunctivitis
- Depression
- Diarrhea
- Dizziness
- Ear infections
- Eczema
- Exhaustion
- Facial swelling
- Flaking scalp
- Fluid retention
- Genital infections or irritation
- Growth of excess body hair
- Headache
- Hives
- Increased hair loss
- Lightheadedness
- Nausea
- Pounding heartbeat
- Redness of skin
- Runny nose
- Sexual dysfunction
- Skin irritation or other allergic reactions
- Vision changes
- Vomiting
- Weight gain

Scalp irritations and cardiovascular disease will increase the absorption of Rogaine, as well as increasing the risk of developing side effects. Systemic side effects can also result from using too much of the lotion.

The standard formulation of minoxidil is a 2-percent solution. Dr. Oppenheim advises that this formulation be used for one year. If results are not satisfactory at the end of that time, he recommends obtaining a special prescription for a 5-percent solution. So medicine's pet "cure" for baldness involves using a powerful drug every day of your life, and upping the dose if it doesn't do the job. When we consider the cost—about $100 per month—and the overwhelming number of possible side effects of using minoxidil on an ongoing basis, plus the nutrient depletion resulting from the use of drugs, there is certainly ample reason to look for a natural alternative. Understand that although minoxidil is rubbed into the skin, rather than ingested, it still gets into the bloodstream very efficiently. The fact that it is applied topically makes it no less toxic. Any drug that must be used indefinitely is obviously not correcting the cause of the problem and so cannot properly be called a cure.

Hair transplants represent an optional way to replace lost hair. This is actually a surgical procedure that can be quite costly and painful. There is also the risk of infection and the disadvantage of living with unsightly scabbing wounds until they heal over. Even the successful hair transplant often looks unnatural, and results can therefore be disappointing. And, once again, nothing is done to correct the cause of the problem.

Nutritional Supplementation

All of the B vitamins are important to the health and growth of the hair. A high potency B-complex tablet (100 milligrams) taken three times daily, with extra amounts of biotin, pantothenic acid, B_6, niacin, and inositol is recommended. Niacin will stimulate circulation, while pantothenic acid, which supports adrenal function, will help offset the effects of stress.

Although iron deficiency can cause hair loss, men should not take supplemental iron unless an iron deficiency is firmly established through laboratory testing because of the dangers of iron overload. (Chapter 6 has guidelines for supplementing with iron.) If you are iron deficient, try taking about 15 milligrams of supplemental iron. Liquid iron tonics seem to be the best absorbed and do not cause constipation.

Vitamin C, taken in 3- to 8-gram doses daily, can aid in improving scalp circulation, as can 90 milligrams of dimethylglycine taken three times daily, and coenzyme Q_{10}, taken three times daily in 60-milligram doses. CoQ_{10} can increase tissue oxygenation. Vitamin E (400 to 1,200 IU daily) is another nutrient that will improve circulation to the scalp through increased oxygen uptake. And 15 to 50 milligrams of zinc and raw thymus glandular can stimulate hair growth by enhancing immune function.

Large doses of vitamin A, exceeding 100,000 international units, taken in the long-term can result in hair loss; however, when the vitamin is discontinued, hair loss stops. Vitamin A treatments, including Accutane, can also cause hair loss.

As constituents of protein, all of the amino acids are needed to maintain healthy hair. Hair and nails each consist of 95- to 98-percent protein. The sulfur-containing amino acids cysteine and methionine are of particular importance. Cysteine is involved in the maintenance of hair strength, supports liver function, and promotes keratin formation. The preferred form of supplemental cysteine is N-acetylcysteine. I recommend taking 500 milligrams twice daily. Sheep given 1 gram per day of cysteine increased their wool production by 14 percent. Also, 500 milligrams of methionine taken twice daily can help prevent hair from falling out. While adequate protein is essential to healthy hair, excess protein can lead to mineral depletion that may cause hair loss.

Essential fatty acids from flaxseed and evening primrose oils are essential to the health of the hair. Deficiency can cause it to become extremely dry and thin, and insufficient EFAs can result in hair loss. I recommend taking one to two tablespoons per day of flaxseed oil with about 50 milligrams of B_6 to assure absorption, plus anywhere from four to six capsules (500 milligrams) of evening primrose oil.

Alternative Treatments

One of the newest and most innovative approaches to stimulating hair growth involves the use of electrical stimulation. In a Canadian study, thirty men received low-powered pulses of electrical stimulation emitted from a device resembling a hooded hair dryer. Such treatment, given twice a week for twelve minutes, resulted in the growth of new hair or the prevention of hair loss in twenty-nine of the subjects. Regrowth of hair occurred in 96.7 percent of the group with no future loss. Such treatment may help to loosen connective tissue that can cause hair follicle strangulation.

In addition to electrical stimulation treatment, I'd like to discuss two other alternative hair loss treatments that have been researched extensively and shown to be effective. First, we have a topical product called Thymu-Skin.* A central ingredient in this product is purified calf thymus extract. Other immune-enhancing ingredients are included in the formula, along with a number of botanicals, such as aloe vera, nettle, and birch. Vitamins A and B and essential fatty acids are also part of the formula.

Thymu-Skin is applied to the scalp twice a day, like minoxidil. Unlike minoxidil, however, its usage tapers off with time. Twice-a-day applications are recommended for four weeks, and then the applications can be reduced to once daily for six to eighteen months, depending upon severity of hair loss. Thereafter, the product can be used every other day and then reduced to twice a week as results dictate. The application of the lotion should be accompanied by a brisk two to three minute massage and hair should be washed twice weekly with Thymu-Skin shampoo.

Studies on Thymu-Skin have been conducted by various prominent researchers, including Dr. Thomas Rabe, a professor in the Department of Gynecology and Endocrinology at the University of Heidelberg, Germany; Dr. M. Hagedorn, a professor at the University of Darmstadt in Germany; and at least a half dozen other notable physicians at reputable clinics in Germany and Vienna. Several of these clinics are for the treatment of cancer, where researchers have established that no hair loss will result from mild or moderate chemotherapy if Thymu-Skin is applied prior to and during treatment.

The exact mode of action of the product is unknown, but it's believed that increased immunity resulting from absorption of the thymus extract through the scalp stimulates follicles to produce tiny new hairs that will eventually grow into terminal hairs. As with most other treatments, Thymu-Skin will not produce new hair growth on those areas of the scalp where hair follicles have died. As long as roots are still intact, hair loss can be stopped and hair growth reactivated. This has been proven in "thousands of patients," according to Dr. M. Hagedorn, who claims that "clinical

---

* Thymu-Skin is available through Yarel biological (1–800–257–5602).

studies on patients who were losing hair caused by alopecia andro-gentica (male pattern baldness) showed that Thymu-Skin treat-ment was successful in 95 percent of the women and 67 percent of the men. Therapeutic success ratios increase with longer periods of treatment."[2]

Another product that has been successfully used in stimulating hair growth is called The Formula.* It evolved out of research con-ducted at the University of Helsinki Medical Hospital in Finland. Researchers noted that shaved laboratory mice to which they had applied a polysorbate-type solution grew hair at a faster rate than did those mice to which no solution was applied. This observation gave birth to a six-year research project on hair growth that culmi-nated in the development of The Formula.

The Formula utilizes a three-step approach to stimulate hair growth. The first step is the cleansing phase, in which the hair fol-licles are cleansed of DHT, sebum, and other clogging secretions. The second step is the washing phase, which includes the use of an all-natural shampoo. This shampoo, with its polysorbate-type ingredients, can be used daily without weakening the hair. Finally, in the activating phase, an activating solution containing twenty-two amino acids is used two to three times per week to nourish the hair. Niacin, which helps improve circulation, is also included in the formula.

Research studies in both Finland and France showed 80 per-cent of those tested experienced positive results. Seventy derma-tologists participated in the French study. The product was found to be safe and effective, and no side effects were reported.

CONSIDER THE FACTS

Male pattern baldness is genetically determined and influenced by the hormone dihydrotestosterone, or DHT. While this condition is by far the most common cause of hair loss in men, it is not, by any means, the only origin. There are several other factors that may be causing your thinning hair, including stress, nutritional deficien-cies, hypothyroidism, drugs, poor circulation, and parasitic infec-tion. These are conditions that you can control. I urge you to con-

* The Formula is available through Nature's Distributors (1–800–624–7114).

sult with a health-care professional who can help you determine the source of your problem.

The cells of hair follicles produce hair when they are supplied with the nutrients they need to stay healthy. In a balding man, these cells aren't receiving essential nourishment, so they die off due to cellular malnutrition. The challenge, then, is to find an effective way to nourish these hair cells. Drugs are not the answer and, in fact, they will likely produce an opposite effect. The best thing you can do is to begin nourishing your body as a whole by eliminating processed foods, choosing quality nutrient-rich foods, and balancing macronutrients.

Supplementing with beneficial nutrients for the hair can also produce good results. These nutrients should include the B vitamins—specifically biotin, PABA, pantothenic acid, and inositol—as well as vitamin E; the minerals iron and zinc; amino acids such as methionine and cysteine; and essential fatty acids.

The best approach to treating hair loss should include the use of both topical applications and a combination of nutrients to nourish you on the inside. No matter which program you decide to follow, however, you should allow up to three months before you expect to see results. And, just to cover all bases, I usually suggest that all my hair-loss clients get an amino acid profile from Aatron (1–800–367–7744).

9.

Overcoming Substance Abuse

Years ago, the words *substance abuse* might have conjured visions of unsavory characters smoking marijuana, shooting heroin, or snorting cocaine. That picture has since changed. Today, many substance abusers are clean-cut, middle-class Americans. And, they're not only abusing illegal street drugs. The fact is, drugs approved by the Food and Drug Administration kill 140,000 people each year—seven times more than heroin, crack, and all other illegal drugs combined. Furthermore, the three most widely used drugs in our culture—caffeine, alcohol, and nicotine—are legal. This is not to downplay the problem we have with street drugs. It's simply to point out that the problem is more far-reaching that most people might think.

Many of my teen clients who abuse cocaine have similar family backgrounds. Dad buys and drinks alcohol by the case and mom routinely takes a half-dozen over-the-counter and prescription drugs to calm her nerves. The entire family has a drug problem, not just the teenager. While some drugs are no doubt more harmful than others, we need to understand that a drug is a drug is a drug. All of these substances are toxic to some degree, and they all rob us of vital nutrients. It's imperative that we strive to keep the use of any drug, no matter how "harmless," to an absolute mini-mum.

While this chapter focuses primarily on alcohol and cocaine, we will also discuss the widespread abuse of cigarettes, marijuana, and coffee. We've all heard about what's wrong with such sub-stances, but we are not often made aware of effective methods for kicking these habits. I will emphasize nutritional solutions that can help you give up these substances with minimal discomfort.

Mainstream advice about overcoming addictions usually cen-ters on mustering up will power, having faith, and/or resolving emotional conflicts. While these are all healthy actions to take, they may be difficult to carry out. They may even be impossible in the face of a powerful, compelling addiction. I use the word "addic-tion" very broadly here; defined as "the experience of being unable to immediately and permanently stop the use of a drug without suffering some degree of discomfort."[1]

The missing component from most drug withdrawal pro-grams—whether it's withdrawal from smoking, alcohol, or illegal drugs—is biochemical repair. The addict can be counseled until the cows come home, but this won't correct the chemical imbalances caused by nutrient deficiencies that perpetuate the condition. Until these imbalances are corrected, no one cannot rightly claim recov-ery—even if abstinence from the formerly abused substance has been achieved. Therefore, much of what has been labeled "recov-ery" is simply the substitution of one addiction for another. Too often, detox involves weaning the addict from his drug of choice, and getting him on another drug or set of drugs. The cocaine addict who trades barbiturates for tranquilizers in the name of treatment isn't cured. He's just started using a more socially ac-ceptable drug. The alcoholic who relies on caffeine, nicotine, and sugar for his highs isn't recovered. Though he no longer drinks alcohol, his body chemistry remains unbalanced. His craving for alcohol and his mood swings and depression are likely to remain. In truth, you can claim to have overcome addiction only when you are no longer dependant upon any harmful substance.

Real recovery is about nourishing your body, freeing it from dependency upon drugs and other damaging substances—including sugar and caffeine—that can be addictive. I believe the negative mental state that gives rise to chemical dependency is itself brought on largely by nutritional deficiency, which is then deepened by drug involvement. Drug therapy for drug addiction may mask symptoms, but it doesn't correct their cause. Replacing missing nutrients can.

An amazingly effective approach to drug and alcohol rehabilitation is one that features nutritional supplements—vitamins, minerals, amino acids, herbs—along with a balanced, wholesome diet to hasten recovery. Coupled with counseling, this is a truly holistic program that helps ease withdrawal symptoms and eliminate cravings. Super nutrition can help you or a loved one kick the habit, whether the addictive substance is alcohol, nicotine, sugar, caffeine, or one of a number of illegal street drugs.

CAFFEINE

Caffeine, in the form of coffee, is the drug of choice for Americans. Collectively, we consume over 400 million cups daily. Statistics show that 50 percent of the population ingests at least two cups of coffee daily, 25 percent take in about five cups every day and the remaining 25 percent drink ten or more cups daily.

Caffeine is an extremely potent stimulant that is widely consumed by Americans, not only in coffee, but in tea, cola, over-the-counter wake-up pills, diet pills, diuretics, cold remedies, and headache remedies. It's similar in effect to amphetamines and cocaine. Chemically, caffeine is classified as a xanthine alkaloid. Other xanthines include theobromine from chocolate and theophylline from tea. All of these substances are similar in their chemical structure and their ability to stimulate the central nervous system. All three are found in coffee.

The caffeine content of coffee depends upon the method used to prepare it. Coffee prepared by the drip method has the highest concentration of caffeine—about 146 milligrams per cup. A cup of percolated coffee has 110 milligrams, while instant coffee has 66 milligrams. And even decaffeinated coffee has some caffeine—about 2 to 5 milligrams—and it often includes traces of the chemical solvent used to remove the caffeine. The most frequently used solvent today is methylene chloride, which can cause irregular or abnormal heartbeat, nausea, and vomiting. A safer solvent, ethyl acetate, is used less frequently. Coffee can also be decaffeinated by the water-process method, which is by far the most preferable technique. However, even when caffeine is removed, oils, acids, tannins, and hundreds of other chemicals remain, many of which also cause physiological changes.

While the amount of caffeine in coffee ranges from 1 percent to 1.3 percent, tea leaves contain 1 percent to 5 percent, depending upon the variety, how the tea is processed, and other factors. The standard cup of tea brewed for five minutes contains 46 milligrams of caffeine; brewed for one minute, it contains only 28 milligrams. Many herbal teas contain no caffeine. Some do, however, so make sure that the label is marked "caffeine free." Be aware that food products such as chocolate also contain caffeine: baking chocolate contains about 35 milligrams per ounce and milk chocolate has about 6 milligrams per ounce. Other caffeine-containing items are listed in Table 9.1 on the facing page.

Ingestion of caffeine, especially in amounts exceeding 200 milligrams, can contribute to many psychological and physiological problems. Included among these are: anxiety; depression; nervousness/irritability; adrenal exhaustion; birth defects; certain forms of cancer (kidney, bladder, ovarian, and pancreatic); diabetes; fibrocystic conditions; heart disease/heart palpitations; high blood pressure; infertility; kidney infection/failure; reduced nutrient assimilation; sleep disorders; ulcers; vision problems (glaucoma); and vitamin and mineral loss.

Many men who drink coffee also smoke. Smokers need to drink a lot more coffee than do nonsmokers to get the same effect. Caffeine stays in a smoker's bloodstream only half as long because the tar in cigarettes increases the rate at which enzymes metabolize it. When the ex-smoker continues to drink coffee at the same rate as when he was smoking, blood levels of caffeine increase dramatically. Tobacco withdrawal symptoms are the same as those caused by high blood levels of caffeine, including anxiety attacks, irritability, nervousness, and sleep disturbance. So when a man stops smoking, unless he also quits drinking coffee—or greatly reduces his caffeine intake—he will have trouble ridding himself of these symptoms.

Table 9.1. Caffeine Content of Common Beverages and OTC Drugs

Beverages	Caffeine (average milligrams)
Dr. Pepper	61
Mountain Dew	55
Tab	49
Pepsi Cola	43
Diet RC Cola	33
Cocoa (1 cup)	13
Diet Rite	32

Over-the-Counter Drugs	Caffeine (average milligrams per tablet)
Bivarin	200
Caffedrine	200
Aqua-ban	100
Excedrin	64
Vanquish	33
Anacin	32
Dristan	16

Caffeine has the effect of constricting blood vessels, which can be an advantage for people who suffer from vascular headaches. For example, individuals who suffer from migraines may benefit from consuming a cup of coffee at the onset of the headache to help relieve it. Because of this analgesic effect, caffeine is often added to pain medications. When a chronic coffee drinker stops, he can develop rebound headaches as a result of the dilation of constricted blood vessels.

Caffeine activates the sympathetic nervous system that governs the fight-or-flight reaction. It also stimulates the brain-altering hormone levels and acts on the pleasure centers of the brain, leading to repeated use. High caffeine intake causes the adrenal glands to continuously secrete adrenaline, leading to adrenal exhaustion and eventually resulting in elevated heart rate and blood pressure, and increased respiration. The liver responds by releasing glucose.

Just as blood sugar rises when we consume carbohydrates, it also rises when we take in caffeine, nicotine, or alcohol. This triggers the insulin response, which can lead to hypoglycemia and, ultimately, diabetes. It also causes the body to store fat. Therefore, in addition to balancing macronutrients, we will need to eliminate, or at least minimize, our intake of these substances to achieve physical and mental balance and weight loss.

Caffeine Withdrawal

Caffeine is a stimulant. So are cocaine, marijuana, speed, and hallucinogens. Brain chemicals called *neurotransmitters* are easily damaged by stimulants, as well as by tranquilizers and other chemicals. These neurotransmitters carry information, in the form of nerve impulses, from the brain to various parts of the body. When drug use damages this relay system, however, the messages aren't always activated properly.

Caffeine, cocaine, and other addictive drugs are thought to produce a "high" by stimulating the production of dopamine. Repeated use of these stimulants can lead to overstimulation and subsequent burnout of dopamine and other neurotransmitters. Amino acids play an important role in repairing damage caused by these drugs because, along with enzymes and other proteins, these protein building blocks make up neurotransmitters. Therefore, tyrosine—a precursor of dopamine, norepinephrine, thyroid hormones, and epinephrine, or adrenaline—can be used as an effective treatment for caffeine withdrawal, as well as for cocaine addiction. The therapeutic effect of tyrosine lies in its ability to replace vital brain chemicals. Tyrosine can be helpful in dealing with the symptoms of caffeine withdrawal. Doses of 1,000 to 2,000 milligrams taken three times daily on an empty stomach about half an hour before meals can help reduce caffeine cravings. Be aware, however, that if you are taking MAO inhibitors for depression, you should not take tyrosine.

Caffeine addiction damages nerve synapses. Withdrawal symptoms—including tiredness, irritability, headaches, and insomnia—can be averted with adequate amounts of the most common neurotransmitter, *acetylcholine*. This brain chemical will repair the nerve-synapse damage. It is manufactured from acetyl coenzyme A and choline, a B vitamin found in fish, liver, eggs, soybeans, peanuts, brewer's yeast, wheat germ, and the lipid lecithin. Five hundred milligrams of choline taken three times daily can help ease the discomfort of caffeine withdrawal.

Dr. Bernard Green, author of *Getting Over Getting High*, suggests that 2,000 milligrams of vitamin B_{12} taken in timed-release form will provide an energy boost and the mental acuity of a cup of coffee in the morning. It should be taken in conjunction with a high-potency B-vitamin tablet or a multivitamin and -mineral supplement that contains all of the B vitamins. Morning exercise can also help energize the body and relieve tension.

In breaking the coffee habit, it's advisable to gradually substitute decaffeinated coffee for regular. Start by making every fourth cup decaffeinated, then every third, and so forth, but do not increase the total number of cups consumed daily. Initially, you should stick with your usual intake. Some people dilute their coffee with more water and less coffee going into each successive cup until finally they're drinking nothing but hot water. You may want to cut back by eliminating one cup every three to four days. Another option is to gradually replace coffee with herb teas, such as valerian or chamomile, or one of the grain-based coffee substitutes, such as Pero or Roma.

Providing the nutritional support your body needs is probably the most important thing you can do. In addition to the B vitamins, vitamin C, calcium, and magnesium can be helpful in combatting stress. Vitamin C will also help detoxify the body. Take 1,000 milligrams extra of vitamin C along with 250 milligrams of B_6 twice daily to help rid your body of the excess liquid that can accumulate when coffee, itself a diuretic, is stopped. The extra intake of vitamins C and B_6 can be discontinued after a few days.

Another antioxidant, vitamin E, can be helpful in large doses of about 800 milligrams on a short-term basis to ease withdrawal symptoms. Choline, vitamin C, and extra calcium and magnesium should be used along with vitamin E for a one-week period following the elimination of coffee from the diet, after which time the dose can be lowered or the supplements discontinued, depending upon your symptoms. There is no harm in continuing these supplements, as well as tyrosine, for as long as needed.

NICOTINE

Whereas caffeine is a stimulant, nicotine is a depressant. Like caffeine, it's a legally available, socially acceptable drug used widely in our culture. Nicotine is our third most popular drug, after coffee and alcohol, although its popularity has decreased somewhat in the last few decades.

Once upon a time it was stylish to smoke. Everyone did it—even doctors. In fact, cigarette advertisements declaring that more doctors smoked Lucky Strike than any other brand appeared in past editions of the *Journal of the American Medical Association.* That changed in 1964, when the Surgeon General's report was issued, confirming the health hazards of smoking including cancer, lung disease, and heart failure. The ensuing campaign against smoking has been surprisingly successful, considering the highly addictive nature of the drug. Per capita cigarette consumption dropped from 4,345 in 1963 to 2,493 in 1994. Back in 1966, 50 percent of the men in this country smoked. By 1988, only 30 percent did.

The fact that smoking is physically addicting was established in 1942, when researchers found that smoker's cravings for cigarettes disappeared following nicotine injections. Today, nicotine patches and chewing gums are widely used to help smokers wean themselves off of this deadly poison. Nicotine's poisonous nature is well known to farmers who use a concentrated spray version of the chemical as a powerful insecticide. Inside the body, nicotine constricts blood vessels, resulting in decreased blood flow to the skin and vital organs.

The toxins in cigarettes are known collectively as "tar." They are byproducts of the combustion of paper, tobacco, and chemicals used in processing. When inhaled into the lungs, this tar causes the air sacs, called alveoli, to lose their elasticity. Ultimately the bronchial tubes and windpipe also lose their elasticity, and emphysema develops.

The major cancer-causing chemical in cigarettes appears to be benzo(a)pyrene. This carcinogenic chemical is also discharged from automobile exhaust and factory smoke stacks. Benzo-(a)pyrene is considered by the American Cancer Society to be a prime cause of lung cancer, the number one killing cancer among men. It's estimated that 75 percent of lung cancer deaths could be avoided if people stopped smoking. Smoking puts men at risk not only for lung cancer, but also for cancers of the kidneys, prostate gland, and bladder.

Nicotine Withdrawal

Anyone who has quit smoking—or tried to—can attest to the fact that it's just not easy. Nicotine addiction is a compelling one. Smokers are hooked just like heroin addicts. But once again, the discomfort of withdrawal can be eased simply by providing the body with nutritional support.

One gram of tyrosine, morning and afternoon, can help stop smoking addiction. Choline, a high-potency B-complex supplement, and vitamin C can all help prevent the cravings associated with nicotine. It's also important to note that smokers have a greater need for vitamin C, since smoking destroys this vital nutrient. This was demonstrated when nicotine was added to human blood and it was found that the ascorbic acid level in the blood dropped 24 to 31 percent.

Vitamin-E supplementation is also crucial for smokers, and for individuals who are trying to quit. Carbon monoxide in cigarette smoke destroys the oxygen-carrying capacity of hemoglobin in the blood.

In addition, smokers have an increased need for vitamin A, because cigarettes lower levels of the vitamin in the respiratory tract. I recommend supplementing with 25,000 international units (IU) of vitamin A for the smoker and aspiring nonsmoker alike.

When giving up cigarettes, it's strongly advised that coffee be eliminated, as well. You've already seen how blood levels of caffeine increase as a result of smoking cessation, thus perpetuating nicotine withdrawal symptoms.

In *Seven Weeks to Sobriety*, author Joan Mathews Larson, Ph.D., observes that successful alcohol rehabilitation depends, in part, on kicking the cigarette habit, because relapse is more common among those who continue smoking. While 25 percent of Americans are smokers, a whopping 83 percent of alcoholics smoke. Dr. Larson advises that, in preparation for quitting, the smoker should set a target date two weeks in the future. During the next two weeks, the smoker should avoid caffeine, junk food, and refined sugars, drink at least six glasses of water daily, exercise every day, and avoid acid-forming foods, such as red meat, organ meats, plums, prunes, and cranberries.

Other nutrients that can help with the withdrawal process include gamma-aminobutyric acid (GABA), glutamine, zinc, and Nicoril capsules. Nicoril contains lobelia and other herbs that the manufacturer (Phyto-Pharmacia of Green Bay, Wisconsin) guarantees will help break the cigarette habit.

GABA is an amino acid that has a powerful calming effect upon the brain. It helps counteract agitation and stress by altering certain neurotransmitters in the brain. Two capsules of Calm Kids by Natrol, with 133 milligrams of GABA per tablet, should be helpful. This product contains several other calming nutrients as well, including glycine, taurine, passionflower, vitamin C, calcium, and magnesium.

Because they are cured with it, cigarettes are composed of up to 75-percent sugar. The amino acid glutamine can serve as an alternative source of glucose to alleviate hypoglycemic reactions among smokers.

Smoking one pack per day of cigarettes deposits 2 to 4 milligrams of cadmium in the lungs, which can lead to emphysema. The body uses a lot of zinc to remove the cadmium buildup. Therefore, smokers are often zinc deficient, and can benefit from an intake of 50 milligrams per day for six weeks.

MARIJUANA

Although marijuana (*Cannabis sativa*) is used by many people for its calming or "mellowing" effects, it's actually a stimulant. Because it's fat soluble, marijuana is stored in the fatty cells of the body and can affect the bloodstream and brain weeks or even months after it's inhaled. Marijuana is slow to leave the body, and therefore it can build up and cause unpredictable reactions.

The major problems associated with the use of marijuana (commonly called "pot") appear to involve its effects upon the mental state. These include apathy, dullness, and lethargy. Emotions and desires become suppressed, and short-term memory and learning ability are impaired.

There does appear to be some benefit associated with the use of organically grown marijuana. Its efficacy in treating visual disorders has been upheld in court and there is some evidence that it may possess properties that prevent cancer. However, if cannabis is not grown organically, nitrosamines can form when it combines with the chemicals in many fertilizers. Nitrosamines are major cancer-causing agents. Harm can also come from the psychoactive ingredients used to cut street pot. It is not uncommon for the pot sold on the streets to contain 4 to 6 percent of these ingredients. There are also some extremely potent hybrid forms of marijuana, such as sinsemilla. With 13-percent psychoactive ingredients, it can lead to hallucinations and emotional problems.

The tar content in marijuana is believed to be equivalent to that of cigarettes. Pot smoking can therefore create the same physical problems as cigarette smoking. Additionally, smoking pot can create age lines and puffiness around the eyes and mouth. Men who smoke several joints daily on a consistent basis often have decreased sperm counts. And, like caffeine and nicotine, marijuana increases blood glucose levels, triggering the insulin response. The short-term problems associated with the use of this drug can be corrected simply by discontinuing its use. It's only with long-term use that recovery may be impaired.

Marijuana Withdrawal

The nerve damage caused by long-term use of marijuana can be repaired by supplementing with choline, taken in doses of 500 milligrams, three times daily, along with a high-potency B-complex formula. Vitamin C (1 gram) is also recommended, as it helps strengthen the adrenal glands and blood vessel walls. Heavy pot users can also benefit from the addition of 500 milligrams each of pantothenic acid (vitamin B_5) and vitamin B_6. Zinc is also important for individuals withdrawing from marijuana because, together with vitamin C, it can chelate cadmium, preventing its absorption.

When eliminating any stimulant from the body, norepinephrine is a critical factor. The amino acid phenylalanine gives rise to tyrosine, which is a precursor to both norepinephrine and dopamine. When phenylalanine is not present in the proteins consumed, depression can result. It's wise to select phenylalanine-rich foods when withdrawing from marijuana, or from any other drug, for that matter. These foods include turkey, cottage cheese, flounder, and roasted peanuts. Adequate phenylalanine intake helps suppress the appetite when small amounts are taken about a half an hour before meals.

Finally, exercise should always be part of any drug-withdrawal regimen. At least thirty minutes a day of physical activity will help produce those "feel-good" endorphins.

COCAINE

Cocaine has become increasingly popular in our culture in recent years. This is indeed unfortunate because its effects can be a danger to users and to the nonusers with whom they associate. A primary danger of this drug is that a person's reaction to it is totally unpredictable. One person may become ill, another temporarily psychotic, and a third may suffer a heart attack from the stimulation cocaine provides.

Cocaine has a fascinating history. Up until 1914 it was actually used in soft drinks. That's right—Coca Cola once had real cocaine in it! And Sigmund Freud was a heavy user of cocaine, as well as a major proponent of its use. He did not, however, consider it to be either safe or predictable.

While some people are able to simply use cocaine, others end up abusing it. The difference between the user and the abuser seems to lie in the efficiency with which their bodies metabolize oxygen. Research indicates that users are normal metabolizers, while abusers have insufficient oxygen flow to the brain, which they seek to increase through the oxygen-like rush to the brain cells that the drug provides. The oxygen starvation that the abuser experiences causes him to feel depressed. That feeling is counteracted by the adrenal rush that cocaine produces.

Cocaine stimulates the sympathetic nervous system, mimicking the nerve reaction to an emergency situation. It blocks the transmission of nerve impulses, instead holding them in the synaptic gap between the nerves. This keeps the nervous system switched on, using the body's reserves of blood sugar and other nutrients for a "quick rush." In this way, cocaine, more than any other stimulant, creates nutritional deficiencies. The damage that the drug incurs on the nerve synapses will make it difficult for the user to think objectively. He may experience hallucinations, anxiety, and personality disorders. Cocaine also causes the body to become dehydrated, especially when it's used in conjunction with alcohol or marijuana.

Cocaine causes an increase in heart rate. When this occurs, oxygen consumption also increases. Pure oxygen will not, however, produce the same high, because it does not increase blood glucose levels, as does cocaine. Some of cocaine's effects, which may vary in degree of severity, are listed below.

- Circulatory system failure
- Muscle twitching
- Convulsions
- Nausea and vomiting

- Cyanosis of the skin
- Feelings of apprehension
- Increased pulse and blood pressure
- Increased respiration
- Loss of muscle reflexes

- Paralysis
- Radical mood changes
- Respiratory failure
- Unconsciousness/loss of vital functions

And the most severe consequence of cocaine use is, of course, death.

Cocaine use increases the concentration of norepinephrine, also called noradrenaline, at the nerve synapse. The result is that the body is pushed into a higher state of metabolism. Consequently, more free radicals are generated. This can lead to the development of degenerative-disease conditions.

Some of the substances with which cocaine is cut—such as tetracaine, butacine, lidocaine, PCP, and methedrine—can be as dangerous, or even more so, than the cocaine itself. Withdrawal programs must be designed to offset the effects of these adulterants, in addition to cocaine. In *Getting Off Cocaine*, Michael Weiner, Ph.D., outlines a thirty-day program designed to break the addiction.[2] The next section covers the highlights of this program and a few suggestions of my own.

Cocaine Withdrawal

Michael Weiner recommends a high-protein diet combined with specific amino acids to repair nerve synapse damage and give a natural energy boost, while taking the edge off the agitation caused by the cocaine. These amino acids, as well as specific vitamins and minerals used in his program, are associated with brain metabolism. The program is designed to increase blood and oxygen supply to the brain, stabilize blood sugar, and provide antioxidant protection. In addition to a multivitamin and -mineral supplement, it incorporates the following elements:

- Adrenal extract
- Calcium/magnesium
- Cysteine
- Dimethylglycine (DMG)
- Glutamine
- Gotu kola
- Lecithin
- Passionflower
- Phenylalanine
- Selenium
- Sudafed
- Tryptophan
- Tyrosine
- Vitamin B complex
- Vitamin C
- Vitamin E

I've already discussed the important functions of several of these nutrients, but let's briefly review a few of them here.

Adrenal extract combats adrenal exhaustion caused by cocaine. This kind of exhaustion is characterized by low blood sugar, fatigue, lethargy, depression, irritability, inability to concentrate, weakness, and poor appetite.

Calcium and magnesium work together to help eliminate muscle cramping and twitching. They are known to be natural tranquilizers and muscle relaxants.

Dimethylglycine (DMG) is an amino acid that improves oxygen utilization at the cellular level, combats fatigue, and increases endurance.

Glutamine is the only substance, other than glucose, that can serve as fuel for the brain. This amino acid helps improve intelligence, fight fatigue and depression, and control cravings for sugar and alcohol.

Lecithin is a lipid that's needed by every cell in the human body. This nutrient contains choline from which the neurotransmitter acetylcholine is derived. Acetylcholine is responsible for nerve transmission, and it regulates the activity of the muscles, and is required for memory, appetite, sexual behavior, and the ability to sleep. Choline and lecithin can have an antidepressant effect and help to combat physical restlessness.

The amino acid phenylalanine is a precursor of tyrosine. It creates a natural feeling of well-being, aids in overcoming depression, increases mental alertness, improves memory, and helps suppress appetite.

The mineral selenium is an antioxidant that protects against free radicals. Its presence is required to activate vitamin E.

Tyrosine is an amino acid that's derived from phenylalanine, and is involved in the manufacture of adrenaline, noradrenaline, dopamine, and thyroid hormones. It also helps overcome depression, increase mental alertness, and improve memory. In a cocaine-detoxification program conducted at Columbia University in New York, investigators reported that 75 to 80 percent of those treated with tyrosine were able to stop cocaine use completely or decrease their use by at least 50 percent.

The B complex vitamins are a team that work together to help combat depression, fatigue, and weakness, and to defend the body against the ravages of stress.

Vitamin C is an important antioxidant that offsets free-radical damage and helps preserve the antioxidant nutrient vitamin E. It plays a key role in the production of neurotransmitters in the brain, helps soothe anxiety and insomnia, and supports the adrenal glands.

Vitamin E is a powerful antioxidant that facilitates oxygen utilization, calms the nervous system, and restores function of a damaged liver.

We have not yet discussed the other supplements listed on page 173. Now, let's take a closer look at some of these important nutrients.

Cysteine, a sulfur-containing amino acid, helps destroy harmful chemicals in the body, such as acetylaldehyde and the free radicals produced by smoking, drinking, and the body's everyday metabolic processes. It protects the body against the effects of radiation, heavy metals, and other harmful substances.

Gotu kola is an herb that has sedative properties. It's also a tonic herb that can strengthen and energize the brain.

Passiflora (passionflower) is another sedative herb. One type of passionflower, Giant Granadilla, has been found to contain serotonin. It helps to calm the body by promoting transmission of subtle nerve impulses, and is useful in combating insomnia, nervous tension, fatigue, and muscle spasms.

Sudafed is an over-the-counter synthetic version of the Chinese herb, ma haung (ephedra), which is useful in treating allergies. The drug stimulates the central nervous system without raising blood sugar. It's similar pharmacologically to cocaine, except the stimulation from it lasts a few hours instead of just a few minutes, as with cocaine. Weiner recommends that Sudafed be used during the first few days of withdrawal from cocaine or amphetamines. He emphasizes the importance of reading the cautions on the label and not exceeding one 30-milligram tablet twice daily, and recommends that it not be taken more than five days without consulting a physician.

The amino acid tryptophan was included in Weiner's program before the FDA prohibited its manufacture and sale in the fall of 1989, following the discovery of a contaminated batch. Prior to that time, it was used successfully in drug and alcohol rehabilitation programs with no ill effects. Tryptophan helps to offset depression by increasing levels of the neurotransmitter serotonin. It has an anti-anxiety effect and helps combat insomnia. While the ban on tryptophan is in effect, one should not attempt to obtain it. Instead, 6 milligrams of melatonin can be used in its place to help induce sleep. Inositol, a B vitamin found in lecithin, is beneficial, as well.

In addition to the supplements and over-the-counter products listed above, Dr. Weiner emphasizes the importance of consuming foods high in phenylalanine to facilitate noradrenaline production. He also recommends avoiding high-carbohydrate meals because they will "slow you down and make you drowsy." That's good advice. People withdrawing from cocaine who experience hallucinations should also use niacin and extra vitamin C. The use of aloe vera or an herbal ointment with vitamin E or goldenseal is good for soothing nasal tissue irritation.

Dr. Weiner also promotes daily exercise—fifteen to twenty minutes per day to oxygenate the system—and the use of coffee enemas to detoxify the body. The caffeine in the coffee stimulates the liver and colon and, absorbed into the portal system, coffee can help flush out the bile in the liver, lightening its toxic load. The same results are not achieved by drinking coffee, due to chemical changes that occur in the stomach. To prepare the enema, boil four heaping tablespoons of ground coffee in two cups of water for ten minutes. Dilute with cold water to make $1^1/_2$ to 2 quarts, and adjust the temperature as needed. Pour into an enema bag.

I believe that Dr. Weiner's recommendations are excellent, though I'd advise doing without the Sudafed, if possible. I also recommend trying some herbs not mentioned by him that can help detoxify the liver and digestive tract. These are listed below:

- Burdock root is a strong liver purifier that also helps balance hormones.

- Dandelion increases the flow of bile, purifies the blood, and is specific for hypoglycemia.

- Ginkgo biloba can be useful in supporting the nervous system. It improves cellular glucose uptake, enhances short-term memory, boosts energy, and is a free-radical scavenger.

- Goldenseal is a liver and blood detoxifier and natural antibiotic that helps reverse liver damage and treat a variety of infections.

- Milk thistle is effective in treating cirrhosis, chronic hepatitis, and alcohol-induced fatty liver. This herb protects the liver cells from damage by environmental and internal toxins.

In addition, the use of enzymes and acidophilus in any withdrawal program can enhance its effectiveness. Acidophilus provides "friendly" intestinal flora that help to digest food and control pathogenic yeast, bacteria, viruses, and parasites. Enzymes assist in the digestive process.

ALCOHOL

Alcoholism is the third leading cause of death in the United States. Relapse is common among alcoholics. Nearly 80 percent of people who receive traditional treatment relapse within two years. Most alcoholics today do not recover. They die prematurely from alcohol-induced disease.

One of the most comprehensive and sound alcohol rehabilitation programs I've encountered is described in *Seven Weeks to Sobriety* by Joan Mathews Larson.[3] Dr. Larson, Director of Health Recovery Center (HRC) in Minneapolis, Minnesota, earned her Ph.D., in part, by compiling the data presented in her book, which is a skillful blend of nutritional research, practical application, personal insight, and a do-it-yourself rehabilitation program.

Dr. Larson's personal insight was facilitated by a personal tragedy that drove her to understand the causes of alcoholism and to seek out effective treatment methods. Years before she became involved in the world of rehabilitation, Larson was suddenly widowed and left with three children. Shortly after her husband's untimely death, her middle child began exhibiting mood swings that were found to result from alcohol-induced hypoglycemia. Despite being given the best of care and treatment over the next several years, her son committed suicide in his senior year of high school.

Larson's search for answers led to her theory that physical rehabilitation is the missing link in the treatment of alcoholism. To test the theory, she founded the Health Recovery Center in 1981. As of 1992, when *Seven Weeks to Sobriety* was published, over three-quarters of the more than 1,000 alcoholics and drug addicts treated there were successfully rehabilitated. This is extremely impressive, since the typical success rate of alcohol rehabilitation is only 25 percent. Today, HRC provides a working model of a holistic approach to rehabilitation—one that incorporates other aspects of treatment such as counseling, but emphasizes biochemical repair of the damage caused by drug and alcohol-induced nutritional imbalances and deficiencies. Much of the information offered here is based upon Dr. Larson's compilation of research data and its application at HRC.

Dr. Larson accurately observes that most addicts have one or more of the following problems:

- Allergies
- Candidiasis
- Heavy metal toxicity

- Hypoglycemia
- Nutrient deficiency
- Thyroid disorders

To get someone off alcohol—or any other drug for that matter—and fail to treat these underlying disorders is a predictable prelude to failure. The above conditions have many symptoms that may masquerade as psychological problems. Therefore, counseling is traditionally used as a primary treatment modality. While it can be an important adjunct therapy, counseling alone will do nothing to correct the above disorders because they are all rooted in physical imbalances.

Of the conditions listed above, I have already discussed hypothyroidism (see Chapter 8) and touched upon problems caused by heavy metals. There seems to be evidence that a buildup of lead and cadmium in the body can predispose an individual to alcohol addiction. Hypoglycemia can be caused by alcohol consumption because alcohol triggers the insulin response. It can also be brought on by excess consumption of sugar and caffeine and aggravated by alcohol. Following the 40/30/30 eating plan can help individuals with low blood sugar to effectively regulate their hypoglycemia.

Now, let's explore the two remaining conditions: candidiasis and allergies.

Candidiasis

Candida albicans is a yeast organism that normally populates the gastrointestinal (GI) tract without causing problems. Several factors can, however, cause candida to change into its fungal form and proliferate in the GI tract and elsewhere, causing a range of symptoms. The body systems most sensitive to the yeast are the gastrointestinal and genitourinary tracts and the endocrine, nervous, and immune systems. Symptoms of candidiasis may include gastrointestinal disturbances such as altered bowel function, bloating, and gas; psychological problems, including depression, irritability, and inability to concentrate; low energy levels; chemical sensitivities; and allergies.

According to Dr. Larson, analysis of the medical records of 213 patients treated at HRC showed that 55 percent of the women and 35 percent of the men had case histories that indicated probable candida overgrowth.

Candida overgrowth is caused by many factors. Chief among them is antibiotic therapy. By destroying all bacteria in the GI tract—the helpful and the harmful—antibiotics reduce the body's immunity and pave the way for proliferation of candida. Refined carbohydrates, steroids, coffee, fluoridated and chlorinated water, and mercury toxicity can also contribute to candida overgrowth by destroying beneficial bacteria in the intestines.

In treating candidiasis, the aforementioned substances must be avoided, as well as foods with a high content of yeast or molds, including alcoholic beverages, cheeses, dried fruits, and peanuts. Refined sugars should also be eliminated from the diet, as well as dairy products (due to their trace levels of antibiotics) and all known allergens. Vegetables, proteins, and whole grains may be included regularly in the diet, however.

Allergies

In listing allergies among the factors associated with alcoholism, Dr. Larson refers to both food and chemical sensitivities. She states that 56 percent of the clients at HRC were found to be sensitive to chemicals in the environment. The most common allergens are ethanol, which is contained in alcohols; automobile exhaust; certain hand lotions and perfumes; gasoline; hydrocarbons; natural gas; tobacco smoke; and soft plastics. Exposure to any of these substances, as well as other chemicals, can trigger intense and sudden responses of anger or sorrow, and cause fatigue, exhaustion, spaciness, mental confusion, depression, cravings, and/or irritability.

Many men have occupational exposure to chemicals. House painters, garage mechanics, hair stylists, and printers, among others, breathe in chemical fumes on the job. Individuals in these occupations are often alcoholic, according to Larson. They become intoxicated by the fumes from their jobs. After a day at work, they are drawn to drink alcohol to stave off withdrawal symptoms. Attempts to stop drinking are foiled by strong cravings for alcohol.

It was the work of allergist Theron Randolph, M.D., that first made us aware of the link between environmental chemical sensitivity and many physical and emotional disorders. Special sublingual allergy testing, in which a sample of the chemical is placed under the tongue, can reveal chemical sensitivities. This testing is done by a clinical ecologist/allergist who is trained not only to identify such allergies, but to desensitize patients to the offending substances.*

While clinical ecologists can test for the food allergies that trigger the same sort of reactions as environmental chemicals, there are some techniques you can apply on your own to identify problem foods. The foods most under suspicion are those you most frequently consume. Wheat, milk, and corn are common allergens for many people. One technique for identifying food allergens is the pulse test. First, establish a regular, resting pulse rate by taking your pulse several times throughout the day and recording it for one full minute. Once you've established your average daily pulse, take your pulse after eating a single food. Take it at five minutes and twenty-five minutes after eating. A pulse twelve or more beats per minute faster or slower than your norm indicates an allergic reaction. Once you have identified the allergen, you should eliminate that food from your diet for the next six months to a year, then rotate it back in, eating it at intervals of four to seven days, but not daily. A similar rotation of tolerated foods can help prevent formation of new allergies and control existing ones.

An important thing to understand about food allergies or intolerances is that, in order for allergies to occur, there must be an excess of "bad" series-2 eicosanoids present. As you'll recall, this excess results from consuming too many carbohydrates. Also, too much alcohol, caffeine, and/or saturated fats will have the same effect. By adopting the 40/30/30 eating plan and eliminating caffeine and alcohol, you can prevent food allergies.

---

* To locate a clinical ecologist in your area, contact the American Academy of Environmental Medicine (303–622–9755).

Alcohol Detoxification

Detoxification is just the beginning of biochemical repair, but it is an important beginning. The following supplements are included in Dr. Larson's detox formula, plus dose per capsule:

Calcium/magnesium	300/150 milligrams
DL-phenylalanine	500 milligrams
Evening primrose oil	500 milligrams
Glutamine	500 milligrams
Mixed amino acids	750 milligrams
Pancreatic enzymes	425 milligrams
Vitamin C	100 milligrams

In addition, Dr. Larson recommends taking a quality multivitamin and -mineral supplement.

From previous discussions, you're familiar with each of these, except perhaps the DL form of phenylalanine. Most amino acids are used just in their L form. I've already described the effects of L-phenylalanine: I just left off the "L." By adding the D to the L form, we get the added effect of pain control and mood elevation through increased endorphin production.

In Dr. Larson's seven-week program, week one is devoted to assessing the damage done by drugs or alcohol. Breaking the addiction begins in week two. That's where detoxification comes in. Dr. Larson actually gives two versions of this detox formula. They differ only in terms of nutrient doses. In both cases, multiple capsules are taken nine times daily. A person's alcohol biotype is what determines the version of the detox formula he will take. (For details on the doses of Larson's detox formulas and additional nutrients used in the remaining five weeks of treatment, I refer you to her book.)

Alcohol Biotypes

Dr. Larson identifies three basic alcohol biotypes. Of these three, the two most common are allergic/addicted alcoholic chemistry and omega-6-EFA deficient alcoholic chemistry.

Dr. Theron Randolph, father of clinical ecology, first put forth the theory that the allergic/addicted alcoholic is actually allergic to alcohol. Dr. Randolph's work has shown that addiction to food and alcohol can produce alternating highs and lows. The occurrence of these up-and downswings depends upon whether the addictive substance is present or absent.

Randolph found that many alcoholics are allergic/addicted to the sugars, grapes, and grains from which alcohol is produced. His findings are substantiated by those of Herbert Karolus, M.D., who found that the majority of the 422 alcoholics he studied were allergic to wheat or rye, the grains that form the base of many distilled liquors. The allergic reaction can effect any organ of the body and can disrupt brain chemistry, altering moods and behavior. The allergic/addicted individual will invariably become ill the first time he consumes alcohol, but with repeated consumption, his body adapts. In fact, the appeal of the alcohol lies in the body's reaction to it. As an adaptive response to the alcohol (or any other allergen), the body will produce endorphins, which create a feeling of euphoria. The endorphin effect is followed by the unpleasant sensations of withdrawal, which drive the individual to resume drinking. Over time, the withdrawal symptoms become more intense and last longer than the high.

Allergic/addicted individuals tend to become angry, depressed, or abusive when drinking—a result of the allergic response of their brains and central nervous systems. They also tend to be binge drinkers and are prone to suffering from hangovers.

Depression is characteristic of the omega-6-EFA deficient alcoholic. Apparently, this depression stems from a genetic abnormality in the way essential fatty acids are metabolized. Normally, they are converted into specific prostaglandins, such as El and PGE1, which prevent depression, hyperexcitability, and convulsions. However, with this biotype, the conversion process is defective, resulting in abnormally low levels of prostaglandin PGE1—a deficiency that causes depression.

When a person with this type of body chemistry drinks alcohol, PGE1 is activated in the brain, which replaces the depression with a feeling of well-being. However, since the brain is hampered in its ability to make new PGE1, the supply of this prostaglandin is gradually depleted. As a result, over time, alcohol seems to lose its ability to relieve the depression.

Because it has gamma-linolenic acid (GLA), evening primrose oil can help the brain convert essential fatty acids to PGE1. GLA is an omega-6 EFA, and a vitally important nutrient for this particular biotype—one that can be identified not only by low EFA levels, but also by ancestry and family history. The omega-6 EFA-deficient alcoholic typically has at least one grandparent who is Welsh, Irish, Scottish, Scandinavian, or Native American. He will generally have a long history of depression and a close relative who was either depressed or schizophrenic. There also may be a family history of eczema, cystic fibrosis, premenstrual syndrome (PMS), diabetes, irritable bowel syndrome (IBS), or benign breast disease. Genetic history influences tolerance to alcohol in the same way it influences food tolerances.

People from the Mediterranean areas of Europe have been drinking alcohol for more than 7,000 years. Today, they have a very low susceptibility to alcoholism—10 percent. Those from Northern European countries, including Ireland, Scotland, Wales, northern parts of Russia and Poland, and the Scandinavian countries have been drinking alcohol for only 1,500 years. As a result, their susceptibility to alcoholism is measurably higher, at about 20 to 40 percent. Native Americans, including Eskimos, had no access to alcohol until 300 years ago, and their vulnerability to alcoholism is extraordinarily high—80 to 90 percent.[4]

Dr. Larson relates a study conducted in Scotland where David Horrobin, M.D., worked with two groups of alcoholics whose EFA levels were 50 percent below normal. One group was given EFA replacement, and the other received a placebo, or "dummy pill," with no active ingredients. The EFA replacement group exhibited far fewer withdrawal symptoms than the placebo group and, three months later, their liver function was almost normal, while there was no significant improvement seen in the liver function of the placebo group. A year later, only 28 percent of the placebo group remained sober, while 83 percent of the EFA replacement group remained sober—and free of depression.

LOOKING TO THE FUTURE

The most commonly abused substances in our culture are caffeine, alcohol, and nicotine, in that order. Although these are legal substances, they are no less toxic than illegal drugs such as marijuana and cocaine. And addictions to all of these drugs can be powerful and extremely difficult to break. But many others have done it, and you can too—you just have to know where to start.

As I said earlier, recovery means no longer being addicted to any damaging substances. It doesn't mean trading alcohol for caffeine or cocaine for tranquilizers. People with addictive chemistries usually use multiple drugs. Traditional rehabilitation programs typically focus on counseling and neglect physical rehabilitation. Often, this sets the substance abuser up for failure because the therapy does not correct the underlying imbalance. True rehabilitation involves nutrient saturation, biochemical repair, and withdrawal from all drugs. And the elimination of processed foods and incorporation of a balanced diet based on the 40/30/30 plan should be an integral part of your withdrawal and maintenance program.

Orthomolecular physicians specialize in a nutritional approach to treating various health disorders. Should you require professional assistance in breaking an addiction, I suggest you contact the Huxley Institute for Biosocial Research at 1–800–847–3802. They can provide you with a list of orthomolecular physicians in your area. You may also wish to contact Aatron (1–800–367–7744) to be tested for amino acid levels and directed to a specific formula based on your individual needs.

10.

Getting in Shape

J ust like making the commitment to eating right, adopting a regular exercise program can change your life. A combination of balanced eating and exercise contributes to a leaner, healthier body. If you are one of the guys who exercises regularly, then you are already reaping the awesome benefits of improved health and increased longevity. What may surprise you is just how much of an impact exercise can have in this regard. Men who exercise reduce their risk of death from all causes by 70 percent, and their risk of heart attack by 39 percent.

In addition to physical health, regular exercise has an enormous impact on mental and emotional well-being. All of you couch potatoes out there will be blown away by the connection between physical fitness and improved mental performance. There are so many good reasons to make exercise an integral part of your daily regimen. The only thing left is to just do it.

Ever hear the saying, "If you want something done, ask a busy person to do it"? Busy people do seem to get more accomplished, including fitting exercise into their crowded schedules. Two-thirds of all American CEOs exercise at least three times per week, while the unemployed are among those who tend to be inactive. Presumably, an unemployed man has more time to exercise than a CEO. And while the excuses of not having the means to join a health club or spa are handy, he can always take up walking, stretching, running, or any number of other exercises that he can do at home without special equipment.

Once the tried and failed excuses of lack of time and money are eliminated, you can begin to focus on finding the type of exercise that's right for you. Men can find clues about what activity they're best suited for in their metabolic rate and blood type, as well as in their personal preferences and current physical condition.

THE MANY BENEFITS OF EXERCISE

The innumerable benefits of exercise should be enough to convince anyone to take up the challenge. Here's a sampling of just a few of them:

- Better digestion
- Control of blood sugar levels
- Elimination of depression
- Enhanced immunity
- Enhanced metabolic rate
- Improved appetite
- Improved eliminations
- Increased circulation
- Increased confidence
- Increased flexibility
- Increased oxygenation
- Increased self-esteem
- Lowered blood pressure
- Lowered cholesterol
- Regulation of the glandular system
- Regulation of insulin production
- Stress reduction
- Stronger bones and muscles
- Toning of the cardiovascular system

The cardiovascular system is favorably affected by the increased circulation resulting from exercise. During physical activity, blood vessels dilate, supplying more blood to the muscles. During vigorous exercise, circulation to the muscles may increase by as much as twenty-fold. According to fitness expert Joanie

Greggains, star of the nationally syndicated TV show, *Morning Stretch*:

> *The heart is the strongest muscle in your body. It's about as big as your fist—and has a big job to do every minute of your life. This is one muscle you want to keep strong. The stronger it is, the more efficient it is at pumping more blood around your body and delivering more oxygen and nutrients to your muscles. This translates into more energy, endurance for your physical health and well-being.*

A fit heart is more more muscular, and therefore more efficient—it beats fewer times per minute at work and when you're resting. When you engage in regular exercise, your heart becomes more powerful, and your pulse rate goes down as the amount of blood pumped by your heart increases. And, finally, your heart becomes stronger, and your arteries become larger to allow for increased blood flow.

Exercise increases not only vascular circulation, but lymphatic circulation as well. The lymphatic system is the body's pumping system designed to eliminate toxins from the cells. It's also an important part of the immune system, because lymphocytes— white blood cells that protect the body from invaders—are formed in lymph nodes, and lymph fluid serves as a carrier medium for these immune cells. Lymphatic congestion or stagnation that results from inactivity has a negative impact on the body's ability to defend itself. Since deep breathing, as well as physical activity, stimulates lymph flow, vigorous exercise can be especially effective in accelerating detoxification and building immunity in the body. This is a major reason why athletes are less prone to develop degenerative disease than people who do not exercise regularly. While one out of three people in our culture will develop cancer, only one out of seven athletes will.

However, the scenario is different for people who overexercise. Dr. Kenneth Cooper, founder and President of the Cooper Aerobics Center in Dallas, Texas, warns that exercise can indeed be a problem if it is excessive. He began observing that professional athletes such as iron man competitors and marathon runners were developing deadly cancers like melanoma and brain tumors. And his friend Jim Fixx, author of *The Complete Book of Jogging*, died of a heart attack while jogging.

Dr. Cooper linked excessive exercise to increased production of free radicals that can eventually break down or destroy the immune system. He recommends moderating exercise and taking a good antioxidant supplement to fight oxidative damage by free radicals.

While strenuous exercise may be contraindicated for some men because of physical limitations, most men can engage in moderate exercise and increase its benefits by integrating deep breathing in rhythm with the exercise. Exercise can have the net effect of lowering blood pressure. Though systolic pressure, which is generated as the heart muscle contracts, can climb as high as 180 or 190 during activity, diastolic pressure shouldn't change. If this happens, it may indicate heart disease.

Exercise can help lower cholesterol. In men, this seems to occur largely through raising beneficial HDL levels. A study conducted in February 1995 involving 2,906 healthy, middle-aged, nonsmoking male runners showed that there was a gradual increase in HDL cholesterol when more miles were run.[1] Most of the changes were associated with distances of seven to fourteen miles per week. Jogging beyond that distance proved to be unnecessary and even counterproductive, due to the increased risk of injury. Using this study as a guideline, we may assume that the man who jogs two to three miles three to four times per week is favorably affecting his cholesterol levels.

Furthermore, exercise also stimulates the glandular system, which aids in the production of neurotransmitters, the brain chemicals that pass messages from cell to cell. Certain drugs—prescription and nonprescription—such as those discussed in Chapter 9, alter the chemical balance in the body by affecting neurotransmitters. We've already seen how specific amino acids can help restore the balance. Well, so can exercise. Like cocaine, exercise is a stimulant that increases norepinephrine levels. However, unlike cocaine, it does not cause nervousness, but instead has a calming effect because of the influence of other neurotransmitters. And exercise increases endorphin levels, which decreases pain and enhances pleasure.

Because physical activity alters blood chemistry, it affects the mind. It influences mental performance, reflecting the balance of neurotransmitters. Mental functioning and emotional state can be adversely affected by minute changes in norepinephrine, acetyl-choline, dopamine, epinephrine, serotonin, and the endorphins. Just a few minutes of vigorous physical activity, however, can restore energy and mental alertness by stimulating norepineph-nine production. Because serotonin and endorphin levels rise simultaneously, stress and depression are alleviated and nervous-ness does not result. So, if you find yourself "brain locked" in the midst of trying to perform a mental task, or if you're too depressed to concentrate, take time out to stimulate your mind by working your muscles. Jump rope, do stretching exercises, or run in place for five or ten minutes instead of taking a coffee break. It will provide the same mental lift, but without the subsequent let down.

PERSONALIZING AN EXERCISE REGIMEN

Generally speaking, men who turn food into energy at a slow rate—the "slow burners" that you learned about in Chapter 2—will benefit most from fast-paced exercise, such as running, cycling, and other aerobic activities that stimulate their metabolism. Fast burners, on the other hand, are better off with exercise that will not stress and deplete their systems, including yoga, swimming, walking, and gardening.

When choosing the best activity for you according to blood type, you should know that men with types B and AB are best suited to milder forms of exercise, as overexertion can lead to exhaustion. If you are one of these two types, choose activities such as yoga, tai chi, and stretching. Individuals with type A blood should also stick with milder forms of exercise, so as not to stress their sensitive immune systems. They would be well suited to activities such as gardening, swimming, light biking, and light weight training. Men with blood type O, on the other hand, will benefit most from vigorous exercises, such as tennis, long-distance biking, and team sports. These activities can help combat fatigue and depression.

If your blood type suggests one type of activity, but your metabolic rate suggests another, you may want to alternate. Try engaging in vigorous activities one day, and less physically stressful exercises the next day.

In addition to making a formal exercise program part of your lifestyle, you should look for opportunities that increase physical activity in the context of your daily routine. For example, try taking the stairs instead of the elevator; choose a parking space a good distance from your destination; walk instead of drive, if possible; walk around the block during your lunch hour or take an exercise break instead of a coffee break to stimulate mental acuity.

Once you have adopted an exercise program, the next important step is to stick with it. As it turns out, 70 percent of people who begin exercise programs quit within one year. Proper nutrition, coupled with an exercise program that's enjoyable, convenient, and appropriate to your personal needs should help keep you motivated. If you find that your program is no longer satisfying or challenging to you, then modify it, change it, or replace it with another program, but do keep the habit of exercise in your lifestyle—for your health's sake.

AEROBIC EXERCISE

Aerobic literally means "with air." Aerobic exercise includes activities that are vigorous enough to make you breathe deeply on a consistent basis for an extended period of time. Aerobic exercise raises the heart rate and works the large muscle groups of the body. This type of exercise is the best way to burn body fat because it reduces insulin levels, provided that the benefits aren't negated by high-carbohydrate intake. After about twenty minutes of aerobic activity, body cells begin releasing fat in the form of fatty acids to be "burned" for energy.

During aerobic exercise, the heart pumps more blood, resulting in increased red blood cell production and improved respiratory efficiency. Engaging in aerobic exercise for thirty minutes four times per week will increase the brain's fuel supply by making glucose more available to the brain. While the average man has 5 million red blood cells in a cubic millimeter of blood, a man who is aerobically conditioned can have almost 8 million. Also, his lungs can become twice as efficient as the average person's.

Aerobic exercise is most beneficial first thing in the morning, when your stores of carbohydrate are low and stored body fat can be accessed. Jogging, brisk walking, rowing, cross-country skiing, bicycling, and jumping rope are all forms of aerobic exercise. There are also structured, choreographed classes available through gymnasiums and health clubs.

In order to build up your cardiovascular system, you must exercise at a minimum of 60 to 75 percent of your maximum heart rate. Maximum heart rate is easy to calculate—just subtract your age from 220. If your goal is to exercise at 65 percent of your maximum heart rate, then take the maximum figure and multiply it by .65. The result is your *target heart rate.* It should match your pulse rate after you engage in vigorous aerobic activity. Pulse should return to normal after three minutes of rest. Advanced aerobic training involves working out at 80 percent or more of your maximum heart rate.

If you are new to aerobic exercise, it's important to start slowly by working out only five to ten minutes at a time and gradually work up to thirty minutes. Jogging two to three miles three to four times per week can bestow cardiovascular benefits by lowering cholesterol. If walking is your preferred exercise, you should start out at 60 percent of your maximum heart rate and work up to 80 percent over a two-month period. Walk at a brisk pace for about an hour three to four times per week. Walking at a pace fast enough to get your heart rate elevated, but comfortable enough to carry on a conversation, is enough to reduce your risk of heart disease by almost 30 percent.

Make sure to warm up by doing five to ten minutes of stretching exercises before walking or jogging. And remember to breathe deeply in rhythm with your steps as you walk. Breathe in through the nose and out through the mouth, inhaling deeply and exhaling fully. When you exhale, you're ridding your body of toxic waste in the form of carbon dioxide.

You may choose to do your walking or jogging on a rebounder. These mini-trampolines provide a flexible jumping surface that minimizes your risk of injury. Due to the spring action of the rebounder, you won't lose energy on the downbounce. Just jumping up and down on the rebounder can provide a good workout and helps to stimulate lymph flow, particularly if paired with deep breathing.

Dr. Phillip Maffetone, trainer/coach for professional athletes, including triathlete champions Mark Allen and Mike Pigg, promotes the 40/30/30 eating plan and advocates training at a relatively low heart rate. According to his formula, you should subtract your age from 180 to obtain the high end of the range and then subtract 10 more to determine the low end. He claims that training in this manner will condition your body to use fat as fuel. Dr. Maffetone subscribes to the idea that aerobic and anaerobic training cannot both be developed at the same time. More information on his approach to fitness can be found in his book *In Fitness and In Health.*

ANAEROBIC EXERCISE

Anaerobic training doesn't aim at raising the heart rate, nor does it make you breathe deeply for an extended period. Because sustained deep breathing is not required, it doesn't build mental stamina in a consistent way, as does aerobic exercise. Strength training through weight lifting is the most popular form of anaerobic exercise among men. This type of exercise increases strength, endurance, and bone density. It improves balance and general overall health. Men of all ages can benefit. Studies have shown that men ranging in age from fifty to ninety-nine not only reaped tremendous benefits from weightlifting, but enjoyed this type of activity. In one study, they worked out only twice a week, performing five exercises of large muscle groups, and still gained the benefits listed above—and they reported feeling much younger.

While weightlifting doesn't call for deep breathing, using proper breathing techniques during exercise will provide added health benefit and help prevent injury. As you lift the weight, breathe out vigorously through your mouth; as you bring the weight down, breathe in fully through your nose.

Research suggests that getting adequate magnesium can actually double your strength benefits from resistance training. It has also been demonstrated that potassium and magnesium aspartate can dramatically improve physical endurance. In 1968, physiologist Bjorn Ahlborg showed that five grains, given in divided doses to six trained athletes increased their endurance on a maximum exercise test by 50 percent! This beneficial effect is thought to result from increased regeneration of adenosine triphosphate (ATP)—the body's primary energy molecule—as well as improved flow of electrolyte transfer across cell membranes.

Because of the tension that builds in strength training, blood flow is impeded, rather than increased. This slows down circulation and causes blood pressure to rise. Therefore, this type of exercise is contraindicated for patients with hypertension or cardiac problems.

BALANCED EATING FOR PEAK PERFORMANCE

Working muscles use more stored glucose in the form of glycogen than inactive muscles. Glycogen stores can become rapidly depleted and the metabolic advantages of exercise quickly lost if the system is overloaded with carbohydrates. When this occurs, the body is unable to regulate insulin production through exercise because it's overruled by the insulin-stimulating effects of the carbohydrates. Therefore, to reap maximum benefits, you should make sure you eat a balanced diet—especially when you exercise.

When someone is in good physical condition we say that he is "fit." Fitness can be measured in terms of oxygen utilization (technically, VO_2 max). Peak performance demands efficient delivery of oxygen to muscles. The rate of that delivery is determined by red blood cells—their number and their thickness or stickiness, known as *viscosity*. This, in turn, is determined by the prostaglandins or eicosanoids generated from essential fatty acids.

The prostaglandin PGE1, vital for treatment of alcoholism resulting from omega-6 EFA deficiency, is also a key to increased athletic performance because it reduces blood viscosity. In this way, PGE1 increases circulation of red blood cells in the capillaries, leading to increased oxygen flow to muscle cells. PGE1 is derived indirectly from gamma-linolenic acid. Taking in enough GLA from evening primrose, borage, and black currant oils can help increase oxygen delivery to the muscles, thereby improving athletic performance. However, if too much red meat is eaten, an overabundance of a certain omega-6 derivative, arachidonic acid, is produced. This substance has a vasoconstrictive effect that can counteract the benefits gained. Clearly, we need to balance our intake of omega-6s, omega-3s, and saturated fats.

But it's not just the consumption of EFAs that determines whether the body will produce "good" series-1 or "bad" series-2 eicosanoids. The production of eicosanoids is also determined by the balance of the macronutrients that we consume. In Chapter 2, you learned how the balanced 40/30/30 eating plan can help you lose weight and build lean muscle mass. Balanced macronutrient consumption creates favorable conditions in which glucagon release, triggered by protein intake, mobilizes body fat. Accessing the body's stored fat for energy spares glycogen, stored in the liver and muscles, making that fuel more available to the brain, stabilizing blood sugar levels, and preserving lean muscle mass. Exercise helps build that muscle mass, and the protein content of a balanced meal helps to sustain it.

However, the typical athlete's diet is composed of 70-percent carbohydrate, 15-percent protein, and 15-percent fat. And the carbohydrates consumed are usually the high-glycemic variety, such as pasta, bread, and potatoes. This type of diet fosters the production of series-2 eicosanoids, precludes the production of PGE1, and impairs athletic performance by decreasing the rate of oxygen delivery to the muscles. In addition, a diet like this will produce constant hunger and decreased mental alertness due to the insulin response and subsequent blood sugar instability it provokes.

Insulin activates an enzyme known as *adipose tissue lipoprotein-lipase* (AT-LPL), which removes fat from the blood and deposits it in fat cells. In this way, insulin acts as a fat-storage hormone. Eating a diet that has the correct balance of macronutrients reduces AT-LPL activity and body fat.

The insulin-reducing benefits of aerobic exercise can be canceled out when you eat (or drink) a high-carbohydrate snack before working out. Under these circumstances, insulin levels will remain elevated, regardless of intensity or duration of exercise. Eaten after the workout, a high-carbohydrate snack will negate the beneficial hormonal benefits that would otherwise have resulted from exercise.

To get the effect he's looking for from carbohydrate loading without *overloading* on carbs, an athlete can instead eat a balanced snack before and after workouts. There are several companies, including The Balance Bar Company, that now make a 40/30/30 nutrition bar. Eating half of a snack with the right macronutrient balance before exercise will assure that the body burns stored fat for energy, rather than carbohydrates, and that good eicosanoids are produced. Eating the other half after exercise helps to maintain the hormonal benefits of the balanced macronutrient intake.[2] Athletes should not consume high-fiber foods, such as whole grains or apples before exercise, because these pull water from the body into the intestinal tract. This impairs performance.

Consuming too much protein in relationship to carbohydrates can actually be worse for an athlete than eating too many carbohydrates, as it can result in the development of *ketosis*, which causes loss of muscle mass. Imbalance in either direction creates problems.

Another benefit of balanced eating is that the higher levels of glucagon, produced by the higher percentage of protein, stimulate the production and utilization of human growth hormone (HGH), which facilitates muscle growth and repair. Series-1 eicosanoids release HGH from the pituitary. On the other hand, excess carbohydrates cause elevated insulin levels, which block hormones that increase production and effectiveness of HGH. Most of the 40/30/30 bars, unlike high-carbohydrate sports bars, contain chromium, which improves the utilization of HGH and amino acids in the cells.

Although the balanced bars are a wonderful aid to athletic performance, remember that you need to maintain the 40/30/30 balance at every meal to continually reap the benefits. I'll show you how to do this in the next chapter. For now, understand that balanced eating improves athletic performance by eliminating hunger; enhancing cardiovascular endurance; eliminating fatigue; increasing muscular endurance; increasing concentration; reducing body fat; increasing oxygen transfer to muscle cells; and improving recovery rate.

According to The Balance Bar Company's President, Richard Lamb, a number of professional and world- and national-class athletes have changed to a more balanced diet modeled after the Balance program with considerable success. Among them are seven medal-winning swimmers in Barcelona; the members of the Subaru-Montgomery professional cycling team; United States pro cycling champion, Bart Bowen; skiers Ewa Twardokens and Robbie Huntoon; national cycling trial champion, John Stenner, and dozens of nationally-ranked triathletes in Southern California.

One study, conducted by the Department of Sports Medicine at Pepperdine University in Malibu, California tested the difference in performance between athletes consuming a diet of 60 percent carbohydrate, 20 percent protein, and 20 percent fat and those consuming the 40/30/30 diet.[3] After four weeks on these different dietary regimens, runners were asked to run four consecutive 5-kilometer segments on a hilly course at training pace, then a final 5-kilometer segment to exhaustion at race pace.

The 40/30/30 group ran significantly faster than the high-carbohydrate group in the last race. They also ran faster in the other segments of the race (though not significantly faster from a statistical point of view) and raised their "good" HDL cholesterol levels by an average of 14 points, when compared with the carbohydrate group. The results of this study indicate that balanced macronutrient consumption increases a competitor's reserve for the final "kick" in competition by enabling him to utilize body fat for energy and spare muscle glycogen. At the end of the study, athletes on the 40/30/30 program reported "better appetite satisfaction, better recovery and better overall feelings of health and well-being."

In another study, published in *Medicine and Science in Sports and Exercise* the running times of six trained athletes were compared on diets with different fat contents: 15 percent (low), 24 percent (normal), and 38 percent (high).[4] It was found that running time to exhaustion was greatest following the high-fat diet (91.2 minutes, compared with 75.8 and 69.3 minutes for the normal and low-fat diets respectively). Oxygen utilization was also higher on the high-fat diet (66.4 ml/kg/minute versus 59.6 and 63.7 for the low-fat and normal diets). While I don't recommend a diet that exceeds 30-percent fat, this study does dramatically demonstrate the performance benefits that can be gained by adding good fat to the diet.

The reason that increasing fat in the diet increases endurance has to do with the fact that fat yields more molecules of ATP than does glucose: Fat yields 460 molecules, compared with 36 molecules from glucose. Also, fat stores in a healthy male adult produce 100,000 kilocalories (calories) of energy, while glucose stores (glycogen) provide only about 2,000.

All of this goes to show that balanced nutrition can be just as important—and very possibly more important—than physical training in shaping an athlete's performance.

MODERATION IS KEY

As you can see, exercise is enormously beneficial to your physical, mental, and emotional health. Some men, however, get carried away pushing their bodies beyond what is healthy. Research shows that an excessive amount of exercise can actually create health problems. Symptoms of overtraining include: apathy, deteriorating performance, diarrhea, elevated resting heart rate, insomnia, irritability, lethargy, loss of appetite, and soreness. While moderate amounts of exercise increase bone density, mineral utilization problems can result from excessive exercise.

Since electrolytes are lost through perspiration during exercise, their replacement is desirable. This is common knowledge among athletes. What many athletes don't know is that some so-called electrolyte formulas lack the critically important trace elements and contain harmful sugar additives that actually leach minerals from the body. Bioavailability of the minerals in such formulas is limited. Instead, use a true electrolyte formula, such as Trace-Lyte, consisting of trace minerals in addition to macro minerals, in crystalloid form, for maximum absorbability.

MAKE A COMMITMENT

Making the commitment to eating a balanced diet is the first step on the road to a healthy lifestyle. Adopting a program of regular, moderate exercise is the next important step—one that can greatly increase your physical and mental performance in your day-to-day activities. Even more astounding are the long-term benefits. Exercise can help you regulate your blood-sugar levels, lower your blood pressure, and decrease your risk of developing heart disease. It keeps your heart beating stronger and longer and strengthens your immune system. In short, exercise can improve the quality of your life.

No one kind of exercise is good for everyone. To reap the greatest benefits, you should personalize your program according to your metabolic rate and blood type. Remember that individuals with blood types A, B, and AB will want to choose milder activities, including yoga, stretching, and light swimming, biking, or weightlifting. Those with type O blood will benefit more from vigorous exercises. And keep in mind that your blood type and metabolic rate may suggest contradictory types of exercise, in which case you'll probably want to alternate between moderate and vigorous exercises.

Finally, don't forget that balanced eating enhances athletic performance, so it's important to maintain a diet approximating the 40/30/30 ratio. Consuming too much carbohydrate before and after exercise can cancel out its benefits.

11.

Super Nutrition at Home

W e're on the brink of a revolution in healthy eating. For the past several years we have been encouraged to consume a high-carbohydrate, low-fat diet for optimum health, endurance, and weight control. We now know that all of these goals can be accomplished on a diet higher in fat and lower in carbohydrates than has been advocated in recent years. The key to reducing body fat is the very same one that unlocks the door to long-lasting energy and stable blood-sugar levels. That key is controlling insulin with macronutrient balance.

As a general rule, the more processed the food, the less fiber it contains—and the worse it is going to be on insulin levels. The sample meals and recipes in this chapter emphasize whole foods that are high in fiber and meals with enough protein to keep insulin's antagonist, glucagon, activated so that you can readily access fat stores. You can lose fat without counting calories.

One of the major problems with the Standard American Diet is that it contains an abundance of bad fats, mostly in their artificial, hydrogenated forms. These fats are hidden in many processed, prepared foods. I'll give you some tips on avoiding these, as well as limiting the friendly saturated fats that can turn into enemies if not balanced with vitally important EFAs and other essential nutrients.

Although I'm more interested in inspiring you to "cut the carbs and add the fat" than to follow the 40/30/30 eating plan to the letter, I offer guidelines below for those wishing to put the plan into action. You'll find an expanded glycemic index in this chapter to help identify those carbohydrates that are converted quickly to blood sugar in the body and therefore trigger a rapid rise in insulin secretion.

CHOOSE YOUR FATS CAREFULLY

By now you know that not all fat is bad. Adequate intake of the essential fatty acids is, in fact, necessary for good health. And, contrary to what we've been told, saturated fats from animal sources and tropical oils are only bad when they're consumed in excess and in the absence of the EFAs and other vital nutrients. Unfortunately, tropical oils, such as coconut and palm kernel oils, acquired a bad reputation as a result of a campaign launched against them in 1986 by the American Soybean Association, which objected to the widespread use of these oils because of the competition that they posed. By the end of 1988, many food companies, responding to consumer fears, began replacing tropical oils with hydrogenated oils. Consequently, coconut oil now accounts for only 1 to 1.3 percent of the U.S. food supply. This is indeed unfortunate because, as you'll remember from Chapter 3, hydrogenation causes harmful trans fatty acids to form.

Coconut oil does not raise blood cholesterol. Instead, it has a neutral effect. Coconut and palm kernel oil have a high percentage of medium chain triglycerides (MCTs). Triglycerides are the chemical forms in which fatty acids occur in vegetable oils. MCTs are easily digested, even for men who have fat malabsorption problems. They stimulate the body's metabolism, thereby aiding in fat-burning. Another advantage of coconut oil is that it contains an antimicrobial component that kills germs.

Both hydrogenated and tropical oils can withstand high temperatures without turning rancid, as do most other oils. They are used in prepared foods such as chips and crackers to increase shelf life. Unfortunately, hydrogenated oils are unhealthy for the human body. Most contain those damaging trans fatty acids, with the exception of hydrogenated tropical oils (see Chapter 3). Although you want to avoid cooking with oils as much as possible—for example, by baking instead of frying)—consider using coconut oil. It is a stable oil that will not turn rancid, or oxidize, easily. Unlike other oils, coconut oil does not need to be refrigerated, since it will remain unspoiled at room temperature for as long as a year.

Olive oil is another good choice. It contains a good balance of fatty acids and is also resistant to oxidation. Flaxseed oil is an excellent source of omega-3 EFAs and contains some linoleic acid, as well. Unlike coconut and olive oil, however, flaxseed oil, as well as other polyunsaturated oils, will oxidize rapidly in the presence of heat, light, and oxygen. Never cook with flaxseed oil, and always keep it refrigerated. The other polyunsaturated oils may be used for cooking, but should always be kept refrigerated.

Trim the (Bad) Fat

While my emphasis has been on cutting carbohydrates rather than fat, I do urge you to eliminate the bad fats and minimize saturated fat in your diet. The September 1994 edition of *Men's Health* magazine ran an article entitled, "50 Ways to Leave Your Blubber" that gave tips on how to cut fats from foods without sacrificing taste. Some of these tips will be useful to you in your quest to reduce your saturated and hydrogenated fat intake. There are also suggestions on how to avoid cooking foods in ways that would expose them to oxidized oils, which can cause free-radical damage.

❑ *Tips for Breakfast*

- Use one instead of two pats of butter on your toast. Never use margarine.

- Instead of regular bacon, substitute Canadian bacon. It has less than half the saturated fat.

- Instead of frying your pancakes, buy the frozen variety and pop them in the toaster.

❑ *Tips for Lunch*

- To avoid the refined oil contained in mayonnaise, either buy it at a health food store or in the specialty section of your local grocery store. Make sure the label says "unrefined" or "expeller-pressed oil"—or try using mustard.

- Instead of using processed mayonnaise in your water-packed tuna sandwich, add lemon, pepper, and hot sauce.

- Choose extra lean or reduced fat ham, which has 3 grams of fat, over regular ham, which has 6 grams.

- If you must have cheese on your sandwich, use grated Parmesan cheese or another variety of hard cheese, rather than cheese slices.

- Use nonfat yogurt mixed with chopped cucumbers and a squeeze of lemon over pita bread stuffed with grilled chicken or beef strips for a low-fat gyro.

❑ *Tips for Dinner*

- Choose lean cuts of red meat—loin and round—rather than rib-eye, which has more than twice as much fat.

- Trim visible fat from meats before cooking them.

- Avoid breaded meat and fish dishes. Breading soaks up cooking oil and seals in fat.

- Heat the skillet before adding oil so less fat will be absorbed by the food. Cold oil soaks into food.

- Cook vegetables in a frying pan or wok with a minimum amount of oil. Start with a small amount and then add water—not more oil—to provide sufficient moisture.

- When eating chicken, choose white meat over dark. Don't eat the skin.

- Use a rack when you roast meat so it doesn't stew in the fat that drips off.

- Try making meat loaf with $^1/_2$ cooked brown rice, $^1/_2$ ground turkey, and $^1/_2$ extra lean ground beef. Top with Worcestershire sauce, barbecue sauce, or ketchup.

- Instead of deep frying your French fries, make oven fries: Slice baking potatoes, sprinkle with cayenne pepper and roast until brown.

- Instead of adding butter to frozen corn, mix the corn with salsa. Add cayenne pepper to the cooking water when preparing corn-on-the-cob.

❑ *Tips for Snacking*

- Choose pretzels instead of chips—but read the label and put those made with hydrogenated vegetable oils back on the shelf. If you must have chips, choose those that are baked, not fried.

- Buy nuts in their shells. They contain less fat, and you'll spend more time shelling and less time eating. Shelled nuts may also become rancid, whereas those still in their shells are protected.

- Make your own tortilla chips by cutting corn tortillas into wedges and baking them on a cookie sheet at 375°F until crisp. Top with salsa.

THE LOW-DOWN ON CONVENIENCE FOODS

Convenience foods include fast foods such as TV dinners. Due to the average American's busy lifestyle, these foods have grown in popularity in recent years, with sales of frozen dinners and entrees doubling between 1982 and 1985. The introduction of the microwave oven was a boon to frozen food sales.

Prepared foods are usually not balanced, nutritious selections. The average frozen-food entree contains over 50-percent fat. Convenience foods also tend to be high in salt and low in fiber. However, some are better than others. And if you find yourself in a position where you must prepare a quick meal, you might want to select a convenience item that is, at least, balanced in macronutrient composition. Table 11.1 lists some convenience foods that conform to the 40/30/30 eating plan.

Of course, Table 11.1 should be used as a guide just to get you started. There are, no doubt, other prepared foods on the market that have the right macronutrient balance. Once again, *read labels.* Besides paying attention to the proportions of macronutrients, look at sugar and salt content and see what additives are in the food. You should rarely rely on convenience foods, but when you must use them, stay as close to all-natural ingredients as possible.

THE GLYCEMIC INDEX

The *glycemic index* is a measure of the effect of carbohydrate on blood glucose levels. It compares blood sugar response after a cer-

Table 11.1. Foods With 40/30/30 Balance

Food	Carbohydrates	Protein	Fat
Prepared Entrees			
Tyson Healthy Portion Herbed Chicken	43 g	32 g	4 g
Swanson's Swiss Steak	36 g	27 g	11 g
Canned Soups			
Progresso's Beef Minestrone	16 g	13 g	5 g
Progresso's Chicken Barley	14 g	10 g	3 g
Progresso's Tomato Beef With Rotini	17 g	12 g	3 g
Healthy Choice Chunky Beef	14 g	10 g	1 g
Campbell's Home Cookin' Beef & Pasta	15 g	11 g	2 g
Campbell's Home Cookin' Vegetable Beef	15 g	11 g	2 g
Chunky Vegetable Beef	15 g	11 g	2 g

tain food is ingested with the body's response after an equivalent amount of pure glucose is ingested. Pure glucose has a 100-percent glycemic index. When you eat any food with a high glycemic index, you will experience a rapid rise in your blood sugar level, which causes your pancreas to secrete a greater amount of insulin. The glycemic index is important because it indicates the effects that different foods will have on blood sugar levels. Many simple sugars, as well as breads and cereals, have high glycemic indexes.

According to the literature published by The Balance Bar Company:

> *The trick to using the glycemic index is knowing when your body needs long-term energy versus a short burst for perform- ance. Before a long workout, a food with a low glycemic index is the best choice because you receive a long, steady release of sugar into the bloodstream. This prevents fatigue and allows you to maintain a steady pace. For intense, intermittent exercise, like basketball, or to rejuvenate your muscles after a vigorous work- out, select a food that is high on the glycemic index scale.*

Table 11.2 is from my book *Beyond Pritikin*. It categorizes some common foods according to their glycemic indexes when com- pared with pure glucose.

Table 11.2. Glycemic Indexes of Selected Common Foods

Glycemic Index	Food
Rapid Inducers of Insulin Secretion	
Greater than 100 percent	Corn Flakes, 40 percent Bran Flakes, French baguette, instant white rice, maltose, millet, Puffed Rice, Puffed Wheat, Rice Krispies, tofu ice-cream substitute, Weetabix
100 percent	Glucose, white bread, whole-wheat bread

Glycemic Index	Food
90–100 percent	Apricots, barley (whole meal), carrots, corn chips, Grape Nuts, Muesli cereal, parsnips, Shredded Wheat
80–90 percent	Banana, brown rice, corn, honey, oat bran, ripe mango, ripe papaya, rolled oats, rye (whole meal), shortbread, white rice, white potato
70–80 percent	All-Bran, buckwheat, kidney beans, oatmeal cookies, wheat (coarse)
Moderate Inducers of Insulin Secretion	
60–70 percent	Apple juice, applesauce, beets, bulgur wheat, couscous, Mars candy bar, macaroni, pinto beans, raisins, rye (pumpernickel), spaghetti (white and whole wheat), wheat kernels
50–60 percent	Barley (coarse), dried white beans, green bananas, lactose, peas (frozen), potato chips, sucrose, yams
40–50 percent	Bran, butter beans, grapes, lima beans, navy beans, orange juice, oranges, peas (dried), rye (whole grain), sponge cake, steel cut oats, sweet potato
Slow Inducers of Insulin Secretion	
30–40 percent	Apples, black-eyed peas, chickpeas, fish sticks (breaded), ice cream, milk (skim and whole), pears, tomato soup, yogurt
20–30 percent	Cherries, fructose, grapefruit, lentils, peaches, plums
10–20 percent	Peanuts, soybeans

40/30/30 MEAL CONSTRUCTION

Super Nutrition is all about balance. So far, you've learned about the importance of eating a moderate diet that is not extremely high in carbohydrate, protein, or fat content. Now you know that it's important to eat according to the 40/30/30 plan—or a modified version of this regimen, according to metabolic rate, blood type, and ancestry. The only thing left is to get started. Don't worry—it's easier than you think!

Below you will find three balanced menu suggestions for breakfast, lunch, and dinner.

Sample Breakfast Menus

Option #1

8 ounces tomato juice
2 poached eggs
2 slices of 7-grain toast (dry)*
$^1/_2$ cup low-fat cottage cheese

* In place of one slice of bread, you may choose one of the following at any meal:
$^3/_4$ cup ready-to-eat unsweetened cereal
$^1/_2$ cup cooked cereal
$^1/_2$ bagel, pita, or English muffin
1 tortilla
$^1/_2$ cup cooked pasta
$^1/_2$ cup cooked rice
$^1/_2$ cup cooked beans
1 small potato (3 ounces)

Option #2

5-egg omelette (1 whole egg, 4 whites)*
$1^1/_2$ cups cooked oatmeal

$^1/_2$ cup skim milk
8 ounces water, decaffeinated coffee, or tea

* In place of 1 medium egg, select one of the items below at any meal:
$^1/_2$ cup creamed cottage cheese or ricotta
1 ounce veal
1 ounce ground beef
4 ounces tofu (soybean curd)

Option #3

6-egg omelette (2 whole eggs, 4 whites) or 1 cup low-fat cottage cheese
2 slices of toast or 2 pancakes
1 piece of fruit* or syrup
8 ounces water, decaffeinated coffee, or tea

* The fruits below have approximately the same number of carbohydrate grams—though they differ in terms of glycemic index rating—and may be used interchangeably:
$^1/_2$ banana
$^1/_2$ cantaloupe
$^1/_2$ grapefruit
15 small grapes
1 small apple, peach, orange, or pear
2 tablespoons raisins
$^1/_2$ cup orange, apple, or grapefruit juice

Sample Lunch Menus

Option #1

4 ounces tempeh with lettuce and tomato
1 whole grain hamburger bun or 1 pita pocket
1 piece of low-glycemic fruit* or salad

Option #2

1 large salad (lettuce, tomatoes, cucumber, etc. with 2 teaspoons dressing)
2 ounces chicken, turkey, seafood, or $2/3$ cup low-fat cottage cheese
1 piece of low-glycemic fruit* or a small roll
1 large sliced apple
Sprinkle with 1 tablespoon granola

*The low-glycemic fruits include:

apples	peaches
grapefruit	pears
grapes	plums
oranges	strawberries

Limit bananas and dried fruits.

Option #3

4 ounces Albacore tuna in water
1 tablespoon canola mayonnaise
2 Ry-crisp crackers
3 cups Romaine lettuce
2 tablespoons fat-free Italian dressing
1 large kiwi

Sample Dinner Menus

Option #1

6 ounces baked or broiled halibut or sole
2 cups cooked low-glycemic vegetables
1 cup cooked pasta or 3 to 4 small red potatoes
1 large dinner salad with 1 tablespoon salad dressing*

* One tablespoon of salad dressing has the same fat value as:

> 1 teaspoon butter
> 5 large or 10 small olives
> 10 large or 20 small peanuts
> 6 whole almonds
> 2 whole walnuts
> 1 tablespoon sunflower seeds
> $1/8$ medium avocado
> 2 teaspoons shredded coconut
> 1 tablespoon cream cheese

Option #2

5 ounces skinned chicken breast or lean beef
1 large baked potato or $1^1/_2$ cups cooked pasta
1 cup cooked low-glycemic vegetables*

* Low-glycemic vegetables include:

artichoke	cauliflower	lettuce
asparagus	celery	spinach
broccoli	cucumber	tomato
Brussels sprouts	eggplant	zucchini
cabbage	green beans	

Limit carrots, corn, and peas.

Option #3

6 ounces soy tempeh for stir fry $1/2$ red or green pepper
1 cup broccoli or snow peas   1 cup cooked brown rice
1 cup zucchini or cabbage

Vegetables that may be substituted for one another, without affecting the carbohydrate balance of the meal include:

$1/2$ cup cooked green beans
$1/2$ medium artichoke
$1/2$ cup cooked asparagus
$1/2$ cup cooked beets
$1/2$ cup cooked summer squash
$1/2$ cup cooked greens
1 cup raw or $1/2$ cup cooked carrots
$1/2$ cup cooked Brussels sprouts

For a low-glycemic dinner, try the following:

4 ounces chicken or lean protein* or 6 ounces fish
3 cups low glycemic vegetables
2 servings fruit (except bananas or dried fruit)

* Lean proteins include:

egg whites   skinned turkey
all fresh and frozen fish   tuna canned in water
lean pork   veal chops and roasts
low-fat cottage cheese   venison
skinned chicken

Snack Options

Choose one of the following snacks when you need a pick-me-up:

1 plain low-fat yogurt
$1/2$ cup low-fat cottage cheese with either 1 apple, 1 orange, 1 pineapple ring, or 2 Ry-Krisp crackers
1 high-protein muffin made with soy or whey protein
1 tablespoon peanut butter on celery

A RECIPE SAMPLER

A nutritious diet that's rich in vitamins and minerals and includes the essential fatty acids is absolutely necessary in maintaining physical and emotional well-being. I have compiled the following recipes to help ease you into your new, healthier eating habits. Each recipe is followed by a breakdown of its carbohydrate, protein, and fat content.

Stuffed Peppers (serves 4)

4 large bell peppers

$1/2$ pound lean ground turkey, uncooked

1 cup of short grain, brown rice

1 medium onion, chopped

$1/2$ teaspoon cayenne pepper

1 teaspoon Italian seasonings

2 cups marinara sauce

1. Preheat the oven to 350°F.

2. Cut opening in top of peppers, clean out interior. Poach peppers in boiling water or steam for 5 minutes.

3. In a separate bowl, mix together turkey, onions, rice, seasonings, and 1 cup of marinara. Stuff each pepper with $1/2$ of the mixture. Place in covered baking dish and bake for 50 to 60 minutes. Pour $1/2$ cup marinara on each stuffed pepper before serving.

NUTRITIONAL FACTS (per serving)

Cal: 270

Protein: 18 g

Carbs: 29 g

Fat: 10 g

Veggie Lasagna (serves 8)

1 pound lasagna noodles, undercooked
2 teaspoons olive oil
2 medium onions, sliced
3 teaspoons Italian seasonings
1 pound sliced mushrooms
2 cups fresh zucchini, sliced
1 package frozen spinach, chopped and thawed
2 tomatoes (24 ounces each), diced
2 cups low-fat Ricotta cheese
2 cloves garlic, minced
$1/2$ cup grated Parmesan cheese

1. Preheat oven at 350°F.

2. In a skillet, heat olive oil, add onions and mushrooms, and cook until onions are soft.

3. Mix in 2 teaspoons Italian seasonings and remove from pan. Set aside.

4. Place zucchini in skillet and saute lightly. Remove and set aside. Add diced tomatoes to onions and mushrooms and simmer for 30 minutes.

5. In a food processor or blender, whip cottage cheese until smooth. Add ricotta cheese and whip together. Add spinach, 1 teaspoon Italian seasonings, garlic, Parmesan cheese, and blend carefully.

6. In a baking dish, layer noodles, cheese mixture, zucchini, noodles, half the sauce, noodles, and remaining sauce. Bake for 1 hour. Let stand for 15 minutes before serving.

NUTRITIONAL FACTS (per serving)

Cal: 240	Carbs: 33 g
Protein: 21 g	Fat: 5 g

Spicy Seafood Casserole (serves 2 to 4)

2 $1/2$ cups cooked brown rice
$3/4$ cup low fat mayonnaise
1 $1/2$ cup low fat milk
1 medium onion chopped
$1/2$ cup chopped green pepper
1 chopped jalapeño
1 clove garlic
1 cup fresh crab meat
1 cup fresh shrimp
1 cup tomato juice
$1/2$ teaspoon cayenne pepper
$1/8$ teaspoon cumin

1. Preheat oven to 350°F.

2. Mix all ingredients together. Place ingredients in lightly buttered or greased 9-x-13-inch casserole dish.

3. Bake for 1 hour. Serve with tossed greens and enjoy!

NUTRITIONAL FACTS (per serving)

Cal: 500	Carbs: 50 g
Protein: 39 g	Fat: 16 g

Cool Pasta Salad (serves 4)

3 cups cooked tricolored rotini, drained and rinsed
2 medium tomatoes, chopped
2 stalks celery, sliced
2 green onions, sliced
2 cups broccoli flowerettes, steamed for 3 to 5 minutes
8 ounces grilled chicken or turkey strips
1 cup vinaigrette dressing
$1/2$ teaspoon crushed basil

1. Combine all ingredients and chill for 2 to 3 hours.

2. Serve on romaine lettuce or lettuce of your choice.

NUTRITIONAL FACTS (per serving)

Cal: 330	Carbs: 37 g
Protein: 25 g	Fat: 10 g

TAKE THE FIRST STEP

Planning balanced, nutritious meals is not such a daunting challenge, once you know where to start. Just base your diet on the 40/30/30 ratio, and modify the plan according to your individual needs. Remember that the secret to regulating your blood-sugar levels and reducing body fat lies in controlling your insulin levels—and that's as simple as taking in the right balance of carbohydrate, fat, and protein.

As you choose your foods, keep in mind that not all fats are bad. You'll want to avoid hydrogenated oils, since hydrogenation give rise to harmful trans fatty acids, and to reduce your intake of saturated fats. On the other hand, you should be sure to include enough of the essential fatty acids in your diet. Try adding supplemental flaxseed oil to your nutritional regimen, since this oil is a great source of omega-3 EFAs and linoleic acid.

Due to the hustle and bustle of the typical American lifestyle, many of us have come to depend on processed convenience foods for sustenance. This is a decidedly unhealthy habit. Packaged and processed foods rarely contain the optimum 40/30/30 balance, and they tend to be high in salt and low in fiber. Plus, convenience foods are generally high in fat—sometimes containing as much as 50 percent! But because it's not always a snap to whip up a meal from scratch, keep an eye out for prepackaged foods, such as those listed in this chapter, that are relatively low in fat and balanced in macronutrient composition.

Finally, emphasize low-glycemic fruits and vegetables in your meal planning. As you learned, the glycemic index rates the effects that certain foods will have on insulin secretion and, therefore, on blood-sugar levels. Foods with a low glycemic index will cause a steady and extended release of sugar into the bloodstream, which helps to regulate blood-sugar levels and prevent fatigue.

12.

Super Nutrition Away From Home

L et's face it—fast food is here to stay. Americans are eating away from home more and more. In 1987, 60 percent of our food dollars were spent eating out. Sales at fast-food restaurants have been increasing by 15 percent every year. Take-out food consumption rose 13 percent in the 1980s, according to a Roper poll. Today's man is no exception—he is super mobile and eats as many as two to three meals in restaurants every day.

You may feel that you simply can't be bothered to deliberate or fuss over food when you're in a hurry. But all you really need is a basic road map to help guide you in making the wisest food selections, including balanced meals that contain a good ratio of carbohydrate, protein, and fat. Healthy meals are built on staples like lean meats, fish, eggs, low fat cheese, vegetables, beans, whole grains, salads, fruit, and natural oils and butter. And you can find most of these foods almost anywhere.

Even still, it can also be a challenge to make fast foods work. Convenience carries with it a price: You can blow your whole daily allotment of calories, fat, and salt at a single fast-food meal if you don't watch what you're eating. However, by learning which food items to avoid and making some simple substitutions, you *can* eat healthy, balanced meals away from home.

THE BASICS

Whether we're talking fast foods or fine dining, the food selection you make can either nourish and sustain you or cause you distress. It's up to you.

One of the biggest challenges in restaurant eating is avoiding the "bad-fat traps," including artery-clogging hydrogenated oils, processed oils, margarine, and fried foods. As we discussed in Chapter 4, you should avoid hydrogenated oils because of the trans fatty acids they contain. These oils are found in foods such as Danish pastries, chocolate chip cookies, muffins, French fries and onion rings, fast-food biscuits, processed cheese, mayonnaise, tartar sauce, and chicken nuggets.

While no one knows for certain how much trans fat the body can tolerate, many experts feel that the daily intake should not exceed 2 grams. The problem is that the most popular fast foods are really top heavy with trans fats. In fact, nutritional expert Dr. Mary Enig found an incredible "8 grams of trans fatty acids in a large order of French fries cooked in partially hydrogenated vegetable oil, 10 grams in a typical serving of fast-food fried chicken or fried fish, and 8 grams in 2 ounces of imitation cheese."[1] Need I say more?

Just remember that the trans fats you're looking to avoid—as well as the saturated ones you want to minimize—may be hiding in creamy, cheesy sauces and dressings, along with plenty of salt and sugar. That's why you want to order these on the side and use them sparingly. Instead of pouring dressing over your salad, try dipping your fork in the dressing before it goes in the salad to minimize your fat intake. Or squeeze lemon over your salad in place of a dressing.

As a rule of thumb, choose those sauces that are wine-based rather than creamed sauces. Likewise, don't make a daily habit of creamed soups—opt instead for tomato, vegetable, or bean so you won't be overloading on certain fats. You'll also want to hold the mayo, and tuna, egg, shrimp, and chicken salads, as well as cole slaw, potato and pasta salads, all of which contain mayo. At home you can use a brand such as Spectrum, which is made with nonhydrogenated oil, like canola. Think in terms of mustard or yogurt instead of commercial mayonnaise. Guacamole, humus (chickpea paste), or salsas, cut with lemon juice, can really satisfy your taste buds and do not contain the trans fat in those mayo-based dips.

The "Fats" of Life

Not all fats are bad, so choose foods that feature healthy or essential fats. Olive oil is a good source of healthy essential fats and is readily available in most restaurants—especially Italian, Greek, and Spanish eateries. A combination of olive oil and vinegar is probably the best salad dressing you can choose use when eating out. Always order the dressing, as well as any sauce, on the side. Use one to two tablespoons per meal. You may drizzle a little bit on your entree, as well as on the salad.

Seafood is a good source of the omega-3 EFAs. You can select from a wide variety of fish and shellfish that are grilled, broiled, poached, or baked in wine and seasoned with garlic and onions. Some Japanese and Chinese dishes use either sesame or peanut oil for stir frying.

A delicious, heart-smart choice offered in Mexican restaurants is guacamole, which contains beneficial monounsaturated fats. It can be used in place of sour cream or cheese as a topping.

A Word About Carbohydrates

When it comes to bread, muffins, crackers, and rolls, try to limit those made with refined white flour—although this is not easy in most fast-food establishments. White flour is a simple carbohydrate rapidly absorbed into the bloodstream. The same goes for pasta, in all of its incarnations. Even though pasta is fat free, it's usually made from white flour. Your best bets, when possible, are whole wheat, rye, or multi-grain. And do remember that sourdough pasta, which may be fat free, is still white and refined.

Enter the Entree

In addition to beans, tempeh, tofu, fish, and poultry for the main protein event, consider veal, beef, and even liver. Men with certain metabolic types—especially fast burners—can handle the heavier meats.

You may want to accompany your entree with a salad, but hold the croutons—they're usually made with hydrogenated oil. Steamed fresh veggies and a potato, brown rice, or corn-on-the-cob with a small amount of real butter are good choices. And do ask if that's really butter on the table. Allow yourself about one pat per meal. Side orders of onions, chives, leeks, and garlic can be added flavor-boosters for your meal.

For breakfast, eggs that are scrambled, poached, or either hard or soft boiled, are a good choice. If you're hankering for whole-grain cereal or fruit, just make sure to have enough protein and good fats at every meal (a scoop of low-fat cottage cheese or a dab of natural peanut butter) so you don't overdo the "crash-and-burn" carbohydrates and go looking for quick pickup from sugar or caffeine in an hour.

FINDING BALANCE IN THE FAST-FOOD LIFESTYLE

It may interest you to know that the following meals provide a pretty good 40/30/30 balance of carbohydrates, protein, and fat:

- The grilled chicken sandwich at Arby's, Dairy Queen, Hardee's, or Carl's (Carbs: 33 g; Protein: 28 g; Fat: 9 g).

- A chicken fajita pita at Jack in the Box (Carbs: 31 g; Protein: 28 g; Fat: 9 g).

- Wendy's chili (Carbs: 29 g; Protein: 24 g; Fat: 8 g) with a few low-sodium crackers.

- A Taco Bell tostada is 30-percent fat. A regular burger from McDonalds is also about the same, but a Big Mac with all the trimmings is more than a whopping 50-percent fat.

Some other fast food items that have the more desirable 30-percent fat content include: baked potato with sour cream; bean burrito; broiled chicken; English muffin; low-fat salad dressing; pancakes; regular shake or malt; and vegetarian pizza. While broiled chicken is 30-percent fat, baked is 35 percent, and fried is 50 percent. The latest bird on the fast-food scene is the rotisserie chicken, touted as a much healthier alternative to fried because fat drips off the chicken when it's rotating on the spit.

Most other fast-food items get over 30 percent of their calories from fat. Some go way over the 30 percent mark. Bacon, for example, and regular salad dressing are 75-percent fat, while cheesecake is 70-percent fat. A taco salad with the shell is 60-percent, as is fried shrimp, fried chicken wings and thighs, a bacon cheeseburger, and an egg and meat croissant.

As far as beverages are concerned, you will want to avoid soft drinks—regular and diet—as their high phosphorus content causes calcium to be leached from the body. You'll do well to avoid or minimize milk and milk-based drinks. Choose bottled mineral water or seltzer, or fruit juices that you can dilute with water. Keep coffee and tea to a minimum because of their caffeine content. Coffee can also cause the body to lose minerals such as calcium, potassium, iron, and zinc, so it's best to avoid it altogether, or drink it between meals. Select herb teas when they're available, but avoid commercial iced tea mixes because they're often presweetened with lots of sugar or aspartame.

SPEAK UP

Make your special needs known to your server. Ask questions when necessary, such as: "Do you serve butter or margarine?" or "What are the ingredients in this dish?" And again, remember to ask for the butter, salad dressing, and sauces on the side.

Don't hesitate to inquire about methods used to prepare foods, and make it clear that you don't want anything fried. You may want to find out what kind of fresh vegetables are available and request to have them steamed when you order them.

Let your server know that you'd like your meal prepared with a minimum of butter or oil and no margarine and that you want to avoid anything containing mayonnaise. Request lean cuts of meat, and don't hesitate to ask the server for his or her suggestions.

ETHNIC CUISINE

While American-style restaurants are the most popular in this country, other favorites include Chinese, French, Italian, Japanese, and Mexican. Middle Eastern, Indian, and Thai restaurants have also become popular, as have those featuring regional cuisine, such as Cajun and Creole. You can order delicious, balanced meals in any of these restaurants.

Chinese

It's real simple when you go Chinese. Just find out what dishes can be made to order and specifically request no MSG, sugar, salt, or soy sauce. You can always add your own soy sauce at the table. If the oil is anything other than peanut, sesame, or canola oil, then order your food steamed. Create combos like beef, chicken, seafood, or tofu with rice and veggies like snow peas, water chestnuts, bean sprouts, broccoli, scallions, bamboo shoots, and bok choy (Chinese cabbage). And try eating with chopsticks. It will probably slow you down and enhance your digestion as a result.

If you go vegetarian, try Buddha's delight, a mix of vegetables and noodles with garlic sauce. You can always add some tofu to these dishes or, if you're not a soy lover, the egg drop soup will add some more protein to your meal.

Lo mein dishes, which are a combination of cellophane noodles (rice or mung bean noodles) with some chicken, beef, shrimp, or other kinds of seafood, are also good choices. Just remember that oyster and black bean sauces are loaded with salt. Try hot mustard, minced garlic, scallions, or Chinese Five Spice powder instead.

Finally, have some green tea with your meal. It's an age-old antioxidant that can also prevent dental caries.

French

Ooh-la-la! You can select from a wide variety of delectable broiled, poached, and steamed foods at French restaurants. Anything sautéed in wine, such as a Bordelaise sauce, is bound to be a winner. The traditional French dish, fish en papillote (cooked with herbs in its own juices) is recommended, as are roast chicken with herbs, steamed mussels, ratatouille (a vegetable casserole), bouillabaisse, and coq au vin. Poached salmon is also a tasty choice, but avoid the heavy butter or cream sauce in this and other selections.

Greek/Mediterranean

Pita bread, also known as pocket bread, is routinely served in these restaurants, along with humus and babaghanoush, two savory vegetarian dips. Humus is a chickpea paté and babaghanoush is eggplant paté. Both are made with sesame butter, garlic, and lemon. Cut with tzatziki (yogurt and cucumber), each can serve as a salad dressing on its own—although the tzatziki alone can do the honors.

You might enjoy a flavorful grain salad, known as tabbouleh, made with bulgur wheat, parsley, onion, tomatoes, olive oil, lemon, and mint. Greek salads and others that feature feta (goat) cheese are also a nutritious choice. Try spinach pie for a satisfying taste treat. And as a main course, you may want to try shish kebab made with grilled meat and vegetables. If you like your food spicy, try souvlaki, a combination of highly seasoned lamb and beef. For a side dish, choose rice-based or wheat-based pilaf known as couscous.

Indian

Indian cuisine features pilafs, rice-based dishes called biryanis, and bean-based dishes known as dals, as well as tandoori chicken and lamb, which are cooked in a clay oven that retains the moisture in the meat. Other tasty entrees include chicken or lamb korma with coriander and yogurt sauce. Curried vegetable and chicken dishes will satisfy those who like spicy foods.

The Indian dahl salad is similar to tabbouleh, made with bulgur, snow peas, and tomato with olive oil. With it you may want to munch on pappadums (lentil wafers) or chapatis and nan (garlic or onion bread). Make sure these are baked, not fried.

Indian cuisine makes liberal use of shredded coconut, coconut oil, and coconut milk. Coconut fat is a healthy saturated fat, which is not harmful as long as it's balanced with EFAs and other essential nutrients.

Italian

It's easy to overload on carbohydrates in the form of pasta, beans, and garlic bread in Italian restaurants. To avoid overdosing, select just one of these delectables. The good news is that you can choose from a wide array of absolutely delicious vegetables, like peppers, zucchini, carrots, cauliflower, and eggplant, that you can't get in a lot of other restaurants. And you can usually select leafy greens, such as spinach or escarole. Sautéed with fresh garlic or onions and a drop of olive oil or chicken broth, these veggies are out of this world.

Then, of course, there are those cheeses—usually mozzarella, ricotta, and provolone. Keep it to a tasty minimum. Try linguine with red clam or mussel sauce, or pasta with chicken or seafood. You can even have your pesto—a sensational combination of garlic, olive oil, basil, pine nuts, and Parmesan—and eat it too. Ask for it on the side. Also, don't overlook the veal dishes, including marsala, piccata, or scaloppini, which are usually quite outstanding in finer Italian restaurants.

Since Italian dishes can be on the oily side, learn to "lemonize" by ordering several lemon wedges that can help emulsify excess oil. And, in your quest to cut down on carbohydrates, have your server take the bread away immediately if you know you're going to indulge in some pasta.

Japanese

As in Chinese cuisine, these dishes tend to feature soy sauce, which should be avoided because of its high salt content. For the same reason, you will need to go light on the teriyaki sauce (a blend of soy sauce, rice wine, and sugar), which is used as a marinade for chicken and beef entrees. Miso, a fermented soybean paste, is also high in salt. It is used mainly as a soup base with sea vegetables.

Japanese restaurants are known for their sushi bars. Choose your sushi with care, as raw fish dishes can be contaminated with parasites. Go for sushi made with cooked crab and shrimp, smoked salmon, and vegetables like avocado and cucumbers.

A good meal starter is tofu-based soup made with kombu or wakame seaweeds. As an entree, try noodle dishes with vegetables and chicken, an assortment of seafoods, fish liked steamed red snapper, grilled salmon or flounder, and some hijiki seaweed with mushrooms and carrots. The sea vegetables featured in Japanese cuisine are rich in trace minerals.

Mexican

Tasty Mexican soups, such as black bean soup and gazpacho, are good choices to start your meal, as is guacamole with lots of fresh lemon or lime juice. You'll probably want to avoid refried beans, because they are generally made with lard—ask to be sure. Corn or flour tortillas are good grain choices, and they can be steamed instead of fried.

You may want to select entrees such as chicken fajitas and chicken or shrimp with rice. Other smart picks include bean, chicken, or seafood burritos or enchiladas, topped with salsa and just a bit of sour cream. But don't overdo the cheese on these dishes because it's a prime source of fat. And, if you're lucky enough to find an authentic Mexican restaurant, squash blossoms, jicama, and chayote cactus are treats for the palate.

Regional Dishes

Tasty, nutritious Cajun and Creole selections include blackened redfish, shrimp or crab boil, chicken gumbo, shrimp Creole, and seafood jambalaya, minus the salt pork used for sautéing and the ham and sausage used for seasoning. Try to keep the meals simple.

SELECTING A RESTAURANT

Aside from personal preference in terms of the type of cuisine selected, there are other factors to consider when you decide where to eat. You may want to select a restaurant that allows you to order a la carte, so that you can control the amount of food you receive. Obviously, you're looking for a restaurant with good quality food—fresh foods, prepared in a healthful manner. You'll also want a pleasant, leisurely atmosphere.

Inspect the menu before being seated if you're unsure of whether or not you can get what you want. And if you have questions, don't be afraid to ask. Shop around for a restaurant that is responsive to your special request—and when you've found it, patronize it regularly and recommend it to others.

ON THE ROAD

Take advantage of the option of ordering special meals when flying on most airlines. These can be provided if they are requested at least twenty-four hours in advance of flight time. Special meals may include fruit, cold seafood, deli, vegetarian, diabetic, and low-calorie and low-cholesterol plates. There is variation between airlines, but all offer some special meals. These meals are often fresher, tastier, and healthier than the standard ones, as they are usually lower in salt, fat, and simple sugars and prepared in smaller numbers.

Try to avoid excessive alcohol consumption when flying, particularly if you're seated in the front of the plane where drinks are free. Limit yourself to a glass of wine with your meal and perhaps an after-dinner drink. Also, make sure that you drink plenty of water when you travel by plane, as dehydration can be a problem due to moisture being withdrawn by the air conditioning system. A good rule of thumb is to drink one glass of water for every half hour in the air. And if you're taking a long flight, you may want to select an aisle seat that offers easy access to the restroom.

Cruise lines will also honor requests for special meals if they are made twenty-four hours in advance of departure time. Perhaps the biggest challenge on a cruise is to avoid overeating, for lavish meals are served pretty much on an ongoing basis. Take advantage of the exercise facilities present on board to walk, run, or swim off the extra calories you may pack away.

When you must spend nights in a town away from home, look for a hotel that has exercise facilities, so that you can keep up with your fitness program. The tendency while traveling is to overeat and to do without exercise. This combination can undo all of the good work you've done at home.

IDEAS TO REMEMBER

Eating away from home doesn't have to mean sacrificing a healthy, balanced diet. You can enjoy a taste-tempting variety of cuisines when you dine out, and still get the right proportions of macronutrients along with an adequate intake of EFAs and other essential nutrients. Plus, by knowing which food items to avoid, you can keep your calorie and salt intake at healthful levels. For example, try to pass on the cream-based sauces, fried foods, and unhealthy hydrogenated fats. Keep your intake of carbohydrates, cheeses, and saturated fats to a minimum. And stay away from ethnic dishes featuring soy sauce, miso, and oyster and black bean sauces, as these are generally quite high in salt content.

Even when you're traveling far from home, you can still maintain your balanced diet. Whether you're taking a plane or relaxing on a cruise, you can request special meals to assure the best available nutrition. Also, take advantage of exercise facilities that are offered in many hotels and on most cruise ships. This way, you don't have to take a break from your exercise program.

Conclusion

Now you know the secrets to improved health and longevity. You're ready to start eating smarter, taking dietary supplements, and shaping up. *Super Nutrition for Men* has shown you how to protect your prostate; keep your heart healthy; combat impotence and infertility; minimize hair loss; and kick dangerous drug habits. You've learned how to choose and maintain the best exercise program for your needs, and you'll be able to select foods that are rich in EFAs, vitamins, and minerals, and low in harmful trans fats, salt, and sugar—both at home and on the go.

So, now that you're easing yourself into a more healthful lifestyle, you can stay healthy and prevent disease by keeping up your appointments with your physician for regular physical exams.

In your twenties and thirties, you should have an annual medical exam. Make sure your doctor orders a complete blood profile that measures cholesterol and high-density lipoprotein (HDL) cholesterol. Also, have your doctor order special screening tests for lipoprotein (a) and iron overload (TIBC and SI). Keep a record of your test results so you can assess your progress.

When you reach your forties, it's time to add a yearly prostate specific antigen (PSA) and a digital rectal exam (DRE). Because I have seen so many men in their fifties who have been diagnosed with prostate cancer, it seems to me that earlier diagnosis might prevent or control this situation. Remember that there are lots of alternatives to the more invasive conventional procedures that involve surgery and radiation. Consider the practice of "watchful waiting," and always get a second or third opinion. After the age of fifty, the addition of a yearly stool test and a sigmoidoscopy every three to five years is helpful to rule out colorectal cancer.

If you travel or back-pack, or if you eat out in ethnic restaurants that specialize in exotic and raw dishes like sushi, I highly recommend that you request the purged stool test from Uni-Key (1–800–888–4353), regardless of your age. This is also a useful screening device to help rule out parasites in unresolved cases of chronic fatigue, irritable bowel syndrome, digestive disturbances, persistent flulike symptoms, arthritic aches and pains, and insomnia.

It's time to take charge and do something about your health. Follow the advice in *Super Nutrition for Men* and you'll see results. You can become a lean, mean, fat-burning machine—and you'll feel better, look better, and enjoy it all because you're healthier.

Notes

Chapter 2

1. Robert Crayhon, *Robert Crayhon's Nutrition Made Simple* (New York, NY: M. Evans and Co., Inc., 1994).

2. Lynne August, "Food and Hormones," *Townsend Letter for Doctors* (April 1995): 56.

3. "She's Lost Weight Eating More and Exercising Less: What's the Secret?" *San Diego Union-Tribune* (Aug. 21, 1994).

4. Hal Walter, "Too Many Carbs!" *Body Talk* (Sept. 1994): 16.

Chapter 3

1. Henry A. Schroeder, *The Trace Elements and Man* (Old Greenwich, CT: The Devin-üdair Company, 1973): 152.

Chapter 4

1. Michael T. Murray, *The Healing Power of Foods* (Rocklin, CA: Prima Publishing, 1993): 35.

2. Gillian Martlew, *Electrolytes: The Spark of Life* (Murdock, FL: Nature's Publishing, Ltd., 1994): 50.

Chapter 5

1. Julian Whitaker, *Health and Healing*, Vol. 2, No. 3 (March 1992): 1.

2. Michael Oppenheim, *The Man's Health Book* (Englewood Cliffs, NJ: Prentice Hall, 1994).

3. G. Champault, J.C. Patel, and A.M. Bonnard, "A Double Blind Trial of an Extract of the Plant Serenoa Repens in Benign

Prostatic Hyperplasia," *British Journal of Clinical Pharmacology* 18 (1984): 461–462.

4. Michael Murray, *The Healing Power of Foods* (Rocklin, CA: Prima Publishing), 333.

5. M.M. Webber, "Selenium prevents the growth stimulatory effects of cadmium on human prostatic epithelium," *Biochemical and Biophysical Research Communication* 127(3) (1985): 871–877.

6. F. Dumrau, "Benign prostatic hyperplasia: Amino acid therapy for symptomatic relief," *American Journal of Geriatrics* 10 (1962): 426–430.

7. Robert H. Phillips, *Coping With Prostate Cancer* (Garden City Park, NY: Avery Publishing Group, 1994), 186.

8. D.T. Wigle, et al. "Mortality study of Canadian male farm operators: Non-Hodgkin's Lymphoma mortality and agricultural practices in Saskatchewan," *Journal of National Cancer Institute* 82: 575–582.

9. M.M. Webber, "Effects of zinc and cadmium on the growth of human prostatic epithelium in vitro," *Nutrition Research* 6 (1986): 35.30.

10. Marsha E. Reichman, et al., "Serum vitamin A and subsequent development of prostate cancer in the First National Health and Nutrition Examination Survey Epidemiologic Follow-up Study," *Cancer Research* 50 (April 15, 1990): 2,311–2,315.

Chapter 6

1. William F. Welles, *The Shocking Truth About Cholesterol* (William F. Welles, D.C. USA, 1990), 41.

2. C.B. Taylor, et al., "Spontaneously Occurring Angiotoxic Derivatives of Cholesterol," *American Journal of Clinical Nutrition* 32 (1979): 40–42.

3. Holden S-H MacRae, "Effects of Low and High Carbohydrate Supplemented Diets on Running Performance," *Sports Medicine Training & Rehabilitation* Vol. 4, No. 4 (1993): 322.

4. *Lancet* Vol. 94 (343): 1454–1459.

5. J. Yudkin, "Dietary Fat & Dietary Sugar in Relation to Ischemic Heart Disease and Diabetes," *Lancet* 2 (1964): 4.

6. J. Salonen, "High Stored Iron Levels Are Associated with Excess Risk of Myocardial Infarction in Eastern Finnish Men," *Circulation* 86 (3) (Sept. 1992): 803–811.

7. Bruce West, *Health Alert* newsletter Vol. 12, Issue 3 (March 1995): 4.

8. Ibid., 5.

9. Julian Whitaker, "Congestive Heart Failure: A New Epidemic," *Health and Healing* newsletter Vol. 5, No. 4 (April 1995): 2.

10. J. Azuma, et al., "Double-blind Randomized Crossover Trial of Taurine in Congestive Heart Failure," *Current Therapeutic Research* 34(4) (1983): 543–557.

11. P.O. Webster and T. Dyckner, "Intracellular Electrolytes in Cardiac Failure," *Acta Medica Scandinavica* 707 (1986): 33–36.

12. Earl Mindell, *Earl Mindell's Joy of Health* newsletter Vol. 3, No. 4 (April 1995), 2–3.

Chapter 7

1. Ming Wei, et al., "Total Cholesterol and High Density Lipoprotein Cholesterol as Important Predictors of Erectile Dysfunction," *American Journal of Epidemiology* 140 (1994): 930–937.

2. William Campbell Douglass, "A Neglected Hormone—Testosterone for Men and Women—Part II," *Dr. William Campbell Douglass' Second Opinion* newsletter Vol. 5, No. 4 (April 1995): 2.

3. Morton Walker, *Sexual Nutrition* (Garden City Park, NY: Avery Publishing Group, 1994), 104.

4. Ibid., 62.

5. M. Costa, et al., "L-Carnitine in Idiopathic Asthenozoospermia: A Multicenter Study," *Andrologia* 26 (1994): 155–159.

6. Walker, op. cit. 92.

7. Ibid., 110.

Chapter 8

1. Morton Walker, "A Hair Raising Tale," *Explore More!* 8 (1994): 44.

2. Michael Oppenheim, *The Man's Health Book* (Englewood Cliffs, NJ: Prentice-Hall, Inc., 1994), 190.

Chapter 9

1. Bernard Green, *Getting Over Getting High* (New York: Quill, 1985), 19.

2. Michael Weiner, *Getting Off Cocaine* (New York, NY: Avon, 1983).

3. Joan Mathews Larson, *Seven Weeks to Sobriety* (New York: Fawcett Columbine, 1992).

4. Ibid., 72–73.

Chapter 10

1. Peter F. Kokkinos, et al., "Miles Run Per Week and High-Density Lipoprotein Cholesterol Levels in Healthy, Middle-Aged men: A Dose-Response Relationship," *Archives of Internal Medicine* 155 (February 27, 1995): 415–420.

2. The Balance Bar Company, promotional literature (Santa Barbara, CA).

3. Holden S-H MacRae, "Effects of Low and High Carbohydrate Supplemented Diets on running Performance," *Sports Medicine Training & Rehabilitation* Vol. 4, No. 4 (1993): 322.

4. Muois, et al., "Effect of Dietary Fat on Metabolic Adjustments to Maximal VO_2 and Endurance on Running," *Medicine and Science in Sports and Exercise* Vol. 4, No. 2 (July 1993).

Chapter 12

1. "Now What? U.S. Study Says Margarine May Be Harmful," *The New York Times* (October 7, 1992): 1.

Appendix A

SUPER NUTRITION MALE MULTIPLE

Here is an example of a daily, broad-spectrum, iron-free formula that can be used alone—for those who are just not vitamin takers—or in conjunction with the other formulas outlined in *Super Nutrition for Men*. Take this formula daily as a supplement to a balanced diet and a healthy lifestyle.

The Super Nutrition Male Multiple contains higher levels of vitamins B_6, B_{12}, and folic acid and is designed to help keep homocysteine levels within a healthy range for better cardiovascular protection.

Nutrient	Dosage
Vitamin A	2,500 IU
Beta-carotene	15,000 IU
Vitamin B_1 (thiamine)	50 mg
Vitamin B_2 (riboflavin)	50 mg
Vitamin B_3 (niacin)	50 mg
Panothenic acid	50 mg
Vitamin B_6 (pyridoxine)	100 mg
Vitamin B_{12} (cyanocobalamin)	1,000 mcg
Biotin	60 mcg
Folic acid	800 mcg
PABA	50 mg
Inositol	50 mg

Nutrient	Dosage
Choline	50 mg
Vitamin C	300 mg
Vitamin D	200 IU
Vitamin E	200 IU
Vitamin K	60 mcg
Calcium	250 mg
Magnesium	250 mg
Potassium	99 mg
Manganese	5 mg
Zinc	25 mg
Boron	1 mg
Copper	1 mg
Chromium	200 mcg
Vanadium	50 mg
Iodine	150 mcg
Molybdenum	25 mcg
Selenium	200 mcg

For the men in my family and for my male clients, I have created a Super Nutrition Male Multiple that is available through Uni-Key (1–800–888–4353). Uni-Key also carries a special biotin product that has helped stop hair loss among my male clients (and it's good for women, too).

Appendix B

SUPER NUTRITION PROSTATE FORMULA

When you decide to undertake a treatment regimen for prostate health, first consider the dietary and supplement recommendations for your specific prostate condition as outlined in Chapter 5.

In addition to an iron-free male multiple supplement, Trace-Lyte electrolytes, and 2 tablespoons of flaxseed oil per day, the following nutrients should be included in your supplemental regimen:

Nutrient	Dosage
Vitamin A	5,000 IU
Vitamin B$_6$ (pyridoxine)	5 mg
Zinc	25 mg
Saw palmetto berry extract	160 mg
Pygeum africanum extract	10 mg
Freeze-dried raw bovine prostate	150 mg

For the men in my family and for my male clients, I have created a Super Nutrition Prostate Formula that is available through Uni-Key (1–800–888–4353). One to two capsules should be taken daily, preferably at breakfast and dinner. Uni-Key also carries a natural progesterone cream for men called ProgestaCare for Men, which can be used in conjunction with the Prostate Formula.

Appendix C

SUPER NUTRITION SEX FORMULA

The following herbal ingredients and nutritional substances provide the safest and most effective natural alternative to Viagra on the market today:

Nutrient	Dosage
Yohimbine	50 mg
Panax ginseng extract	40 mg
Ginkgo biloba leaves extract	20 mg
Saw palmetto berry extract	40 mg
Freeze-dried raw orchic tissue	100 mg
Dimethylglycine (DMG)	90 mg

For the men in my family and for my male clients, I have created a Super Nutrition Sex Formula that is available through Uni-Key (1–800-888–4353). One to two capsules should be taken daily, preferably with breakfast and dinner.

Appendix D

PERFECT FOOD WHOLE-FOOD FORMULA

Even though organic produce is more widely available today than ever before, it can be hard to find in many areas—and it's expensive! But because there's such a quality difference between organic and nutrient-poor commercially-grown produce, you don't want to compromise. Now, no matter what your situation, you don't have to forego organic foods in favor of less expensive commercial foods. A product called Perfect Food is a whole-food powder concentrate that will provide you with the equivalent of ten servings of organically-grown nutrient-rich vegetables and two servings of fruit. This powerful formula is a blend of over fifty whole foods and food complexes in their pure unadulterated forms along with the crucial beneficial soil bacteria normally present in rich, organic soil. The foods have been specially processed, allowing them to retain all of their nutrients. And there are no herbs added, so you can take it every day.

❏ **Defense Greens Complex** contains a blend of kamut grass, barley grass, alfalfa grass, oat grass juices (all 33:1 concentrate), spirulina, chlorella, spinach, broccoli, three-day-old broccoli sprouts, kale, cauliflower, parsley, dandelion, grass, sea kelp, sea dulse, and sea vegetables.

❏ **Defense Concentrated Whole-Food Matrix** is a food-based vitamin and mineral blend. It contains twenty-two naturally occurring amino acids and tocotrienols (forty to sixty times more potent than standard vitamin E as an antioxidant) and over seventy antioxidant compounds. The Whole-Food Matrix also has a twenty-six percent fatty acid content.

❏ **Defense Seed Blend** includes chia seed, flaxseed, and pumpkin seed. Flaxseed is the most potent source of plant lignens ("good" fats) such as omega-3 and omega-6 essential fatty acids. Chia seed is the most nutritious—and expensive—of all seeds. It's packed with EFAs, including omega-3s and -6s, and contains powerful antioxidants and highly digestible proteins.

❏ **Defense Veggie Juice** is a blend of carrot, beet, and tomato juices.

❏ **HSO™ Formula** contains homeostatic soil organisms and resident probiotics in a host of plant-derived minerals and ionic trace elements originating from ancient sea deposits.

❏ **Soy Sprouts** are nearly 40-percent protein and rich in phytochemicals.

❏ **Acerola Extract** is the richest source of vitamin C and bioflavonoids.

❏ *Lactobacillus salivarius/plantarum* **(1 billion CFU per serving)** is a patented prototype lactobacillus strain that is specially designed to digest proteins.

The Perfect Food Whole-Food Formula is available from Uni-Key Health Systems (1–800–888–4353).

Index

Healthy Habits

are easy to come by—

IF YOU KNOW WHERE TO LOOK!

Get the latest information on:

- **better health • diet & weight loss**
- **the latest nutritional supplements**
- **herbal healing • homeopathy and more**

HEALTH BOOK CATALOG

ACHIEVING HEALTH

AVERY PUBLISHING GROUP

1998

COMPLETE AND RETURN THIS CARD RIGHT AWAY!

Where did you purchase this book?

❑ bookstore   ❑ health food store   ❑ pharmacy
❑ supermarket   ❑ other (please specify)_____

Name_____

Street Address_____

City_____State_____Zip_____

RECEIVE A FREE COPY OF AVERY'S HEALTH CATALOG

GIVE ONE TO A FRIEND ...

Healthy Habits

are easy to come by—

IF YOU KNOW WHERE TO LOOK!

Get the latest information on:

- **better health • diet & weight loss**
- **the latest nutritional supplements**
- **herbal healing • homeopathy and more**

HEALTH BOOK CATALOG

ACHIEVING HEALTH

AVERY PUBLISHING GROUP

1998

COMPLETE AND RETURN THIS CARD RIGHT AWAY!

Where did you purchase this book?

❑ bookstore   ❑ health food store   ❑ pharmacy
❑ supermarket   ❑ other (please specify)_____

Name_____

Street Address_____

City_____State_____Zip_____

RECEIVE A FREE COPY OF AVERY'S HEALTH CATALOG

||| ||

Avery Publishing Group

120 Old Broadway
Garden City Park, NY 11040

I..II...III....I.III....I.I.II......II.I.I...II.I

|| | ||

Avery Publishing Group

120 Old Broadway
Garden City Park, NY 11040

I..II..III....I.III....I.I.II......II.I.I...II.I